The Anesthesia
FACT BOOK

The Anesthesia
FACT BOOK

*Everything You Need
to Know Before Surgery*

FRANK SWEENY, M.D.

PERSEUS
PUBLISHING

A Member of the
Perseus Books Group

Library of Congress Control Number: 2003100410
ISBN 0–7382–0823–X

Perseus Publishing is a member of the Perseus Books Group.
Find us on the World Wide Web at http://www.perseuspublishing.com.
Perseus Publishing books are available at special discounts for bulk purchases in the U.S. by corporations, institutions, and other organizations. For more information, please contact the Special Markets Department at the Perseus Books Group, 11 Cambridge Center, Cambridge, MA 02142, or call (800) 255–1514 or (617) 252–5298, or e-mail j.mccrary@perseusbooks.com.

Text design by Jeff Williams
Set in 11-point Minion by the Perseus Books Group

First printing, March 2003

1 2 3 4 5 6 7 8 9 10—06 05 04 03

This book is dedicated to my parents, Patricia Ann and John Paul to whom I owe my life and to my three biggest supporters, Yadi, Sara, and Sydney.

Contents

Acknowledgments

I could not possibly name all the people who have helped to make this book a reality. First, I'd like to thank my agent, Joelle Delbourgo, who believed that patients should have an understandable reference book on anesthesia that answered their common questions.

I also give warmest thanks to my editor at Perseus, Marnie Cochran, who had faith in this project and thought this book would benefit patients. I also thank Marnie for her guidance and patience keeping the voice of this book directed to the audience for whom it was written.

I would like to thank the entire Perseus family for their assistance in getting me whatever was necessary for the completion of the book. I would also like to give special thanks to Ingrid Finstuen, Erin Sprague, and Jon Howard at Perseus, who helped get this manuscript from one electronic media to another.

I must give special thanks to the crack research team in the Burlew Library at St. Joseph's Hospital: Jan Grabowski, Soraya Itan, Ann Ryan, and Julie Smith. Their tireless and amazingly quick literature searches are deeply appreciated.

Lastly, I would like to give special thanks to my busy colleague and friend, Dr. Klane Hales, for his precious time in reading the manuscript and providing valuable input.

Introduction

In the next year, some 40 million people in the United States will undergo a procedure requiring an anesthetic. Some 2,000 or more of these patients will die from causes related to their anesthesia care. Many times this number of patients will suffer from complications related to anesthesia. It is estimated that more than half of these deaths and complications are preventable.

The subject of anesthesia inspires both fear and fascination in most patients. Studies have shown that anesthesia often evokes more fear and anxiety for patients than the surgery for which it is being given. One study on the nature of preoperative anxiety reported that, of the top ten concerns expressed by patients, eight were related to the anesthesia they would receive for the procedure—not the procedure itself! With almost daily stories in the electronic and written media describing disasters associated with anesthesia, patients are more concerned than ever about the potential risks and complications associated with anesthesia for themselves and their loved ones. Patients don't know if these disasters are an incredibly rare event or a daily occurrence. They don't know if they are preventable or inevitable. Patients are unable to distinguish a safe anesthesia caregiver from an unqualified one, a safe operating facility from a dangerous one.

Despite these questions and concerns, patients will meet with their anesthesiologist on average for less than five minutes before surgery. The patient invariably has several questions she would like to discuss with the anesthesiologist. The anesthesiologist, who is inevitably under severe time pressure to keep the operating room on schedule, has precious little time to answer these questions. During this hurried and often unsatisfying meeting, the patient is left with a host of unanswered questions and unresolved anxieties about anesthesia.

Although each patient is unique, her questions are not. In fact, the questions, misconceptions, and fears that patients harbor regarding anesthesia are remarkably consistent. This book will answer 99 percent of the questions that you have about your anesthesia care. It dispels some of the myths associated with anesthesia administration, and it will explain the process of anesthesia administration.

This book exposes grossly substandard practices that occur before, during, and after anesthesia that are still prevalent throughout this country. It will give you the knowledge to identify these practices and how to avoid them. Much of the time anesthesia administration is safe, but there are still outrageous transgressions in standards of care that will put some patient at far higher risk than others. When patients are uninformed about the process of anesthesia, they will take unnecessary risks, and they will suffer needless harm.

As the medical director of one of the busiest operating rooms in California, I decided that I would try to improve the experience of patients coming to surgery by preparing a little pamphlet answering the most common questions patients ask about anesthesia. At the same time, I would improve patients' understanding of the process of anesthesia and the role of the anesthesiologist in their care.

The list of questions was generated from twenty years of clinical anesthesia experience with more than 20,000 patients. I started writing answers that are commonly given to patients that tend to promote surgery and anesthesia, and I realized that I wasn't telling the whole story. In fact, my answers weren't even close to the truth. As I started writing real answers to the questions instead of the comic-book version, the little pamphlet grew. I took my typed answers to the hospital print shop, where they told me I needed a publisher, not a copier. Thus this book was created.

"If a little knowledge is dangerous—where is the man who has so much as to be out of danger?"

—THOMAS HUXLEY

PART I

Before Surgery

1

Who's the Person Giving My Anesthesia? Do Credentials Matter?

The people who administer anesthesia in the United States today are not all equally qualified or equally safe. Before you decide who will do your surgery, who will do your anesthesia and where it will be done, you had better think twice. Then think again. These may be among the most important medical decisions you ever make. You don't want them to be the *last* decisions you ever make. These decisions should not be left strictly to chance. In the words of R.E. Shay, "Depend on the rabbit's foot if you will, but remember it didn't work for the rabbit."

Out of the approximately 40 million patients who received anesthesia in the United States in the past year, a physician specializing in anesthesiology administered less than half of those anesthetics. More than 3 million procedures were performed in doctors' and dentists' offices in 2000. Studies indicate that a physician specializing in anesthesiology was present in the office surgery suite during surgery in less than one-third of these cases.[1]

Most patients assume that their surgeon or dentist has pre-screened the person administering the anesthesia and would not be working with them if they were unqualified. This is a reasonable assumption, but it's often wrong. Patients don't interview and select their anesthesia caregiver in the same way they choose their surgeon or dentist. It's amazing that patients, or the parents of children scheduled for anesthesia, do not routinely ask the qualifications of their anesthesia caregiver, yet the anesthetic is often associated with more risk than the procedure. Patients know far more about the person who cuts their hair than they know about the person who is responsible for keeping them (or their child) safely anesthetized during surgery.

Individuals administering anesthesia in the United States have widely different levels of training, competence, and standards of practice. Studies have demonstrated that the risk of anesthesia is related to the level of training of the person who administers it. The hierarchy of anesthesia caregivers may be grouped into three categories based on their level of education and training in the discipline of anesthesia. Ranked from most highly trained to least trained (or untrained), they are:

1. Physician anesthesiologists
2. Certified registered nurse anesthetists (CRNAs)
3. "The Others"

Physician Anesthesiologists

The most highly trained of all those who administer anesthesia are the physician anesthesiologists, commonly called *M.D. anesthesiologists*. To become an M.D. anesthesiologist, the individual must complete four years of college, four years of medical school, obtain an M.D. degree, complete one year of internship, and then complete a minimum of three years in an accredited residency program in anesthesiology. An optional fifth year of further training, or fellowship, may be taken in one of the subspecialty areas of anesthesiology. Add it all up and you realize that formal postsecondary education required is generally twelve or thirteen years before an M.D. anesthesiologist enters into her specialty.

M.D. anesthesiologists hold unrestricted medical licenses and are trained as physicians first and anesthesiologists second. In medical school and the internship, the prospective anesthesiologist must first learn about all areas of medical practice before specializing in the discipline of anesthesiology.

The first two years of anesthesiology residency are devoted to learning all aspects of clinical anesthesiology. The third year of residency is spent in advanced training in specific areas of anesthesia such as cardiac anesthesia, obstetrics (OB) anesthesia, pain management, pediatric anesthesiology, and so on. Up to one-third of anesthesiology residents will spend an additional fourth year after completing their residency engaged in specialized training (the fellowship). This fellowship year may be spent specializing in cardiac anesthesia, pediatric anesthesia, obstetric anesthesia, pain management, critical care medicine, or perioperative anesthesia.

The scope of anesthesia training for the M.D. anesthesiologist goes far beyond the operating room because the scope of practice of anesthesiology has changed dramatically over the past four decades. Forty years ago, the practice of anesthesiology was almost exclusively limited to the operating room. Today, the duties of an anesthesiologist extend to the preoperative anesthesia clinic, the postanesthesia care unit (PACU), the pain clinic, the intensive care unit, and as administrator and coordinator of the operating room.

A significant portion of the anesthesiology residency program for an M.D. anesthesiologist is spent in perioperative management of the patient. Perioperative management is the care and preparation of the patient before, during, and after the surgical procedure. This is as important as the administration of the anesthetic itself. The anesthesiologist must decide if the patient is in their best medical condition for surgery because this profoundly influences outcome in patients with significant coexisting medical problems. The anesthesiologist also spends a considerable amount of time learning about the management of acute and chronic pain.

At the completion of this training, the physician anesthesiologist may voluntarily sit for the American Board of Anesthesiology exam. This consists of a written exam, which, if passed, is followed by an oral exam. If the oral exam is also passed, the physician becomes a board-certified anesthesiologist. Currently, there are approximately 38,000 M.D. anesthesiologists in the United States.

Certified Registered Nurse Anesthetists

The second most highly trained of all those who administer anesthesia are the certified registered nurse anesthetists. To become a CRNA generally requires four years post–high school to achieve a bachelor of science degree in nursing , a minimum of one year of clinical work in either an intensive care unit setting or a recovery room setting, and then two years in nurse anesthesia school. Some CRNAs will only complete a two-year RN program followed by two years in nurse anesthesia school. Formal postsecondary education required is generally between five and seven years before a CRNA enters into her specialty.

The CRNA's anesthesia training is a combination of classroom and clinical work. Most nurse anesthesia schools offer a master's degree upon completion of the program. Following nurse anesthesia school, the nurse anesthetist may take a qualifying exam, which if passed results in the title certified registered nurse anesthetist.

The duties of the CRNA are generally confined to the operating room administering anesthesia. Medicare rules currently require that a physician or other practitioner with an unrestricted medical license supervise the CRNA in the hospital setting. States vary on their requirements for supervision of CRNAs. The physician supervising the CRNA is most often an M.D. anesthesiologist, but a surgeon, radiologist, or any other physician with an unrestricted medical license may do so. With approximately 28,000 CRNAs, they deliver about half of all anesthetics given in the United States today.

"The Others"

Others who administer anesthesia are by far the least trained and often the least educated group to assume responsibility for administering anesthesia. This diverse group includes any individual who administers anesthesia other than the M.D. anesthesiologist or the CRNA. As unbelievable as it sounds, outside the accredited hospital or ambulatory surgery center setting, the person who administers anesthesia may literally be anyone. It may be an unlicensed office worker, receptionist, office manager, RN, dental hygienist, radiologist, dermatologist, surgeon, or dentist.

"The Others" frequently have had no formal anesthesia training. The average amount of formal training in anesthesia administration of nurses, dental hygienists, and technicians who administer anesthesia is zero. The average amount of formal training in anesthesia administration of nonanesthesiologist physicians is zero. Although dentists may choose to take a few weeks or months of training in the administration of sedative medications and nitrous oxide in dental school, their average amount of time spent in formal training in anesthesia administration is close to zero. Oral surgeons who administer anesthesia generally spend six months to one year in anesthesia training during residency.

Does It Matter Who Administers the Anesthesia?

The topic of who will administer anesthesia to the patient is an emotionally charged issue. At times, it's difficult to discern where the political rhetoric begins and ends and when there is a true patient safety or quality-of-care issue. Each group has its own political, economic, and professional agenda to advance and protect.

Few will argue that "The Others" are relative bottom-feeders in the hierarchy of anesthesia caregivers. This is an extremely diverse group of anesthesia providers who have a striking lack of uniform educational and training standards and a striking lack of uniform adherence to accepted standards of patient care. This group is the most likely to have egregious violations of accepted safety standards, accepted standards of monitoring, and accepted standards of patient care. This group is the most likely to operate in an environment that will shield them from peer review, accrediting agencies (like the Joint Commission on Accreditation of Healthcare Organizations), mandatory reporting of adverse outcomes, and oversight by federal, state, and local laws.

The discrepancy in quality of anesthesia care between M.D. anesthesiologists and CRNAs is less obvious, yet the rancor between the political talking heads representing each group is at times extreme. Both groups have highly trained anesthesia providers who follow accepted safety standards for anesthesia delivery and patient care. CRNAs as a profession have been dedicated to providing quality anesthesia care for more than 100 years and continue to serve crucial needs for anesthesia delivery in undersupplied areas. CRNAs are the sole providers of anesthesia care in about two-thirds of all rural hospitals in the United States. Shortages of anesthesia services exist nationwide, exacerbated by the push for fewer physician specialists and more primary care physicians during the Bill Clinton years. At this time, we need every capable M.D. anesthesiologist and CRNA to cover the existing demands for anesthesia services.

There are several different practice models of anesthesia care delivery in this country today. In some practice models, only M.D. anesthesiologists administer anesthesia. In others, only CRNAs administer anesthesia. The *anesthesia care team* model is a combination of CRNAs and M.D. anesthesiologists working together. Other practice models may be hybrids of the above models. The use of the anesthesia care team model is widespread in this country because of critical anesthesia personnel shortages, cost effectiveness, and in some cases to improve the quality of care. CRNAs in solo practices tend to occur in small facilities like the office-based surgery suite and in more rural areas where procuring an M.D. anesthesiologist is difficult.

The only serious debate among politically active M.D. anesthesiologists and CRNAs is whether CRNAs should be allowed to practice anesthesia *independently* of a physician's direction. This is a point of bitter contention. M.D. anesthesiologists contend that the knowledge base of CRNAs, resulting from less postsecondary education and less advanced clinical anesthesia training, leaves them less capable of providing comprehensive patient care before, during, and after surgery. There are legitimate differences in the amount of postsecondary education and legitimate differences in clinical training between CRNAs and M.D. anesthesiologists as stated above.

Do Credentials Make a
Measurable Difference in Outcome?

Studies of patient outcomes related to different models of anesthesia care delivery and different anesthesia providers have been done. The highest mortality rate was seen with nonspecialists (surgeons and dentists) providing anesthesia. The next highest mortality was seen with CRNAs practicing independently. The M.D. anesthesiologist practicing alone had lower mortality than either of these two groups. However, the M.D. anesthesiologist working with the CRNA in the anesthesia care team model had the lowest mortality of all groups.[2] More recent literature indicates that when a physician anesthesiologist is directing the anesthesia care in an elderly population, the reduction in mortality can be substantial.[3]

The influence of the trained anesthesia specialist extends far beyond direct patient care. Much impetus for implementation of standards of preoperative and postoperative care, improved standards of patient monitoring, critical incident analysis, routine use of recovery rooms, and so on, came about because anesthesia specialists identified risk factors and implemented safety and practice standards to reduce these risks whenever possible.

In the end, there is a great deal of evidence that suggests that it does matter who gives you your anesthesia. Since 1950, the number of physician anesthesiologists in the United States has increased approximately sixfold. At the same time, the mortality associated with anesthesia has dramatically declined. In 1954, a study of mortality associated with anesthesia and surgery reported that deaths directly attributable to anesthesia to be about one in 2,700 patients.[4] In the 1990s, the reported mortality attributable to anesthesia was between one in 20,000[5] to one in 250,000[6] or less, depending on the patient group being studied. The sixfold increase in physician anesthesiologists is largely responsible for this increased safety,[7] although improvements in monitoring, pharmacology, and nursing care during this time period have also contributed heavily.

What You Should Do

What you should do as the patient (or as the parents of the child having anesthesia) is some research in advance. The easiest way to do this research is by asking questions. Regarding your anesthesia caregiver, it is reasonable for you to ask:

- Who will administer my anesthesia and what are his/her qualifications? The answer will tell you a great deal about the quality of the facility where you or your child will have your procedure. If the individual administering the anesthesia has no credentials or training to do so, I would ask for a person who does. If this is not possible, I would reconsider having the procedure done elsewhere.

- Is the individual administering my anesthesia certified by his/her certifying organization? Sometimes it's a warning flag when the individual administering the anesthesia is not certified by his/her own organization. If the person scheduled to administer your anesthesia is not certified, please ask why not.

- When will I meet or speak with the individual responsible for administering my anesthesia? This is important because it gives you the chance, in advance, to determine the qualifications of your anesthesia caregiver. You do not want to be in the holding room immediately prior to surgery to find that an unqualified individual will be administering anesthesia to you or your child. Your surgeon acting as your anesthetist does not necessarily imply competence. If your surgeon claims to be a qualified anesthetist, ask them about the formal training they have received in the administration of anesthesia.

Conclusion

The training and credentials of your anesthesia caregiver do matter. The M.D. anesthesiologist and CRNA are specially trained and highly qualified to administer anesthesia. "The Others" who administer anesthesia are a very diverse group, often with minimal training and dubious credentials. It is important to know the qualifications of your anesthesia caregiver before you give your consent for anesthesia.

2

Will I Speak to My Anesthesiologist Before Surgery? Does It Matter?

In one of the largest studies ever conducted on death attributable to anesthesia, inadequate preparation for the case by the anesthetist was the most common factor.[1] Indeed, inadequate assessment of the patient was cited in more than half of these deaths. This included inadequate preoperative evaluation or inadequate investigation of problems. Almost half the deaths in this study were attributed to inadequate treatment of the patient's coexisting medical problems before surgery. The authors concluded that more than one-fourth of these cases should have been cancelled because the patient was inadequately prepared for surgery. The importance of preoperative evaluation and optimization of the patient cannot be overstated. Only through speaking with your anesthesiologist can such a thorough evaluation be made.

The Purpose of the Meeting Between Anesthesiologist and Patient

Ultimately, the goal of the meeting between you and your anesthesiologist is to make anesthesia and surgery as safe as possible. How do we accomplish this task? First, the anesthesiologist must identify relevant medical history and physical factors that will impact your anesthesia management. The anesthesiologist may glean important information before the case that will make your anesthesia safer and indicate a specific anesthetic technique that should be used or a specific anesthetic technique that should not be used. Second, the anesthesiologist must be certain that you are in your best possible medical condition prior to surgery. This will have the greatest impact on reducing the risk of anesthesia and surgery. How are these goals accomplished?

The history: The anesthesiologist should review all of your relevant medical and anesthesia history that might impact your anesthetic management and identify problems that need further investigation. Your old charts and records should be reviewed whenever possible. The information in them can be lifesaving. It may reveal some salient issue that puts you in jeopardy or suggests certain precautions or preparations that are needed before safely proceeding with your anesthesia. This includes your coexisting medical problems, family history of anesthesia problems, and prior anesthetic experiences. A proper preoperative evaluation identifies the patient who may have a coexisting disease or condition or medication use that could unexpectedly impact the management of anesthesia.

Limited physical exam: Your anesthesiologist should perform a cursory physical exam relevant to anesthesia. Evaluating your airway is essential. Listening to your heart and lungs is advisable as well. Cardiac or pulmonary abnormalities may be detected that may indicate new problems or poorly controlled existing disease.

Preoperative testing: Based on findings in your history and physical exam, the anesthesiologist, primary care doctor, or the surgeon may order lab tests. These lab tests will help determine if you're in your best condition for surgery. If your doctors still have questions about your condition after the history, physical, and lab testing, then it is appropriate for consultation with an appropriate specialist. For example, new and worrisome electrocardiogram (ECG) changes would require consultation with a cardiologist. *Healthy patients frequently require little or no lab testing despite widespread practices to the contrary.*

The anesthesia plan: Following the preoperative medical evaluation described above, your anesthesiologist should discuss the anesthesia plan with you. This plan will take into account the surgery, your preferences, the surgeon's preferences, and the anesthesiologist's preferences. Your safety should always come first. The anesthesia plan includes a discussion of the anesthetic management during surgery, the plans for pain management after surgery, and even your expected length of stay in the hospital. Your informed consent is obtained during this portion of the visit.

The benefits of a good preoperative meeting: The meeting between you and the anesthesiologist may substantially reduce your anxiety. Education should be an important part of this visit and has been shown to increase patient satisfaction, decrease patient anxiety, decrease postoperative pain medicine requirements, and even decrease length of stay in the hospital.[2] Ultimately, the most important reason of all for this meeting is to reduce the morbidity and mortality of surgery and anesthesia.

How Can the Preoperative Evaluation Reduce the Risk Associated with Surgery?

Studies have consistently shown that the preoperative condition of the patient is the most significant predictor of postoperative morbidity and mortality. Less severe manifestations of disease are associated with substantially lower morbidity and mortality during and after surgery. When patients are in their best medical condition coming to surgery, they will have far fewer complications. Studies have consistently demonstrated that when the patient is not in their best medical condition prior to surgery, and their diseases are not well controlled, the risk is several times greater than when the surgery is performed with medical conditions of the patient under good control.[3] For example, in the patient who has chronic congestive heart failure, the risk of surgery and anesthesia may be five times greater if the surgery is done as an emergency and the heart failure is not well controlled prior to surgery.[4] Even a preoperative condition as simple as a common cold will significantly increase your risk of having an airway or lung complication during or after surgery.

Based on the results of your preoperative interview and evaluation, the anesthesiologist must determine if you are in the best medical condition for your planned surgery. If you are in your best medical condition, then surgery proceeds. If you are not in your best medical condition, then the surgery should be postponed, if possible, until you are.

When Should the Meeting Between Patient and Anesthesiologist Occur?

Twenty years ago, most patients were admitted to the hospital the day prior to surgery to have their preoperative evaluation and testing done. The anesthesiologist would visit the patient the night prior to surgery in the hospital room after having reviewed all relevant medical history, test results, and consultant notes, and the anesthesiologist would have a leisurely meeting with the patient. If something was missing or questions raised that required further investigation, it could be addressed the night prior to surgery. This was an ideal—though exorbitantly expensive—way to prepare patients for surgery.

With the realization that many procedures could be performed safely on an outpatient basis (in and out the same day) with tremendous cost savings, everything changed. Currently, 65–70 percent of all surgeries are done as outpatients. Another 20–30 percent are performed as same-day admits (which means you might stay overnight after your surgery, but not before). Even the vast majority of open-heart and brain surgery patients are admitted the morning of surgery. About 5 percent of surgeries are performed in surgeons' offices. Thus, only a very small number of elective surgery patients are admitted to the hospital the night before surgery.

The need for proper preoperative evaluation and preparation of the patient for surgery hasn't changed in the past twenty years, but the logistics of how this occurs has changed dramatically—and it isn't all good news. Most often, the anesthesiologist must accomplish the entire preoperative interview, evaluation, and informed consent process in about five minutes or less! Unless you are completely healthy and have no questions, it is difficult if not impossible to accomplish all the goals of the preoperative visit in this short period.

The standard bedside preoperative visit puts substantial time- and cost-saving pressures on your anesthesiologist to hurry through the process and avoid delays and cancellations. This *production pressure* may put you at risk if your anesthesiologist misses an important piece of information about your condition that should be addressed before surgery, or if there are any questions that should be answered prior to surgery. Your anesthesiologist, in an effort to avoid delays or cancellations, may waive important tests or appropriate consultations that would resolve questions about your fitness prior to surgery.

The objective is to have you in your best possible medical condition coming in for surgery because this will decrease your risk of complications. All questions about your health should be answered prior to surgery. How this is accomplished is less important than the imperative that it must be accomplished. The methods used to accomplish this objective are as varied as the institutions performing surgery. For healthy patients who require little if any testing, the usual abbreviated anesthesia visit five minutes before surgery may be adequate even if it is unsatisfying for both the patient and the anesthesiologist. For the patient who has coexisting diseases, the preoperative evaluation requires considerably more lead time before surgery to be done properly.

If you have coexisting disease, your assessment and testing should occur far enough in advance of your surgery so that your medical diseases can be in their best condition at the time of surgery. Much of this preliminary testing will be arranged and reviewed by your primary doctor and surgeon. This may result in a diagnostic or therapeutic intervention for a specific medical problem that may decrease your risk. A completed workup in advance of surgery also reduces cancellations or delays on the day of surgery.

In some institutions, a specific anesthesia preop and evaluation clinic (APEC) exists for this purpose. In a perfect world, the patient arrives at the APEC, is given a questionnaire about their health, and, based on the results of the assessment and a limited physical examination, would have the indicated tests done at the facility. The results of these tests would be evaluated by a physician who works in the APEC, and based on the results the patient would either be ready for the upcoming surgery or, if any questions remained unanswered, would be scheduled for consultation with the appropriate specialist. The visit to the APEC must occur far enough in advance of surgery that the consultation with the specialist, if needed, would be completed in advance of surgery. Healthy patients would not be required to visit the clinic unless there was some special patient need or desire. In a perfect world, patient education would an important part of this visit.

Conclusion

The importance of a proper preoperative visit with an anesthesiologist cannot be overstated. The greater the number and severity of your medical problems, the more important the meeting is. If you have significant medical problems, you should insist on speaking with an anesthesiologist well in advance of surgery to address any problems, questions, or concerns you have. It will allow time for you to have any additional tests, consultations, or preparations completed and evaluated in advance of surgery that may avoid delays or cancellations on the day of surgery.

Lastly, if your anesthesiologist or surgeon appears to be in a rush or hurrying through this process in the moments before surgery, please ask him to slow down and be careful. "Haste encouraged by situation" has been shown to contribute to accidents and errors in anesthesia.[5] It is time well spent to resolve questions about your fitness for surgery or to answer questions about the most appropriate anesthesia for you. Safety should always come first.

3

Why Do Doctors Order So Many Tests Before Surgery?

Instead of a proper preoperative evaluation and assessment of the patient, many physicians simply order a battery of tests. Dr. George Lundberg, a nationally respected pathologist and former editor of the *Journal of the American Medical Association*, estimates that about 80 percent of all lab tests ordered by physicians are unnecessary.[1] A review of studies on screening preoperative laboratory testing reveals that the vast majority of these tests are of no demonstrable benefit to the patient.[2] A study of preoperative lab testing revealed that two-thirds of all testing in outpatient surgery patients was inappropriate and unnecessary, mostly related to obsolete habits by the physicians ordering the tests.[3]

This does not imply that all lab testing is unnecessary—far from it. The objective of the entire preoperative process is to have you in your best medical condition within the context of your diseases. The purpose of lab testing is to detect an abnormality that may affect anesthesia management or your response to anesthesia and to optimize your medical conditions before surgery.

Unfortunately, many physicians still think good medical care means ordering the greatest number of lab tests. Too many or too few tests are equally undesirable. The best medical practice is to order the indicated tests, no more and no less than are required based on the interview, preoperative history, physical exam, and the magnitude of the planned surgery.

During the 1970s, technological progress in lab testing made it possible to measure up to twenty different lab values simultaneously on a single sample of blood. Patients who were otherwise completely healthy and had no evidence of disease based on their history and physical exam would routinely have their blood analyzed for these twenty different lab values. In addition to blood tests, electrocardiograms and chest X-rays became routine for all patients scheduled for surgery because it was erroneously believed that such tests were useful screening tools to identify those who had unsuspected or unknown diseases.

Anesthesiologists soon learned that batteries of blood tests, ECGs, and chest X-rays were *not* good screening tools for disease in asymptomatic patients. In fact, unless the preoperative history and physical exam suggested a problem, screening lab tests were counterproductive. Normal, healthy patients coming for surgery would have lab abnormalities discovered that were either spurious or clinically insignificant to the patient and to anesthesia management.

It is important to understand the concept of "normal" in lab testing to understand why an "abnormal" result may not be significant. Lab tests have a *reference range* that is defined as "normal." *Normal* is defined as the specific lab test results that will include 95 percent of asymptomatic patients who are subjected to the test. That is, if 100 completely healthy people were to have a lab test, the test results that would include ninety-five of the 100 subjects tested would define the *normal reference range*.

Statistically, even if you are completely healthy, you have a 5 percent chance of falling out of the normal reference range. You have a 2.5 percent chance of being higher than the upper limit of normal, and a 2.5 percent chance of being lower than the lower limit of normal on any given test. An otherwise healthy person whose lab value falls outside the normal reference range is considered abnormal. Is there any clinical significance to this abnormal lab value in an otherwise asymptomatic person? Probably not. Despite this, the abnormal lab test result will either be repeated, investigated, or ignored and considered clinically insignificant. Why would a doctor order a test if he was going to ignore the result if it came back abnormal?

Subjecting patients to batteries of tests is not cost-effective or an efficient way to pick up an unrecognized disease. Studies show that screening tests on asymptomatic and apparently healthy patients do *not* improve the quality of care or the outcome of those patients.[4] Even if the patient does have stable coexisting disease, doctors must consider the magnitude of surgery when deciding on what lab tests are needed before surgery. For example, cataract surgery is minimally invasive to the patient and takes about a half-hour to complete. Eliminating all preoperative lab testing before cataract surgery does not measurably affect the risk of surgery.[5]

In contrast, studies have shown that unnecessary lab testing carries risk to both the patient and the physician ordering them. A study showed that one in 10,000 asymptomatic patients *may* receive some minor benefit from a screening chest X-ray. These benefits were not lifesaving discoveries. However, one in 2,000 preop chest X-rays leads to unnecessary *patient harm* from pursuit of a clinically insignificant abnormality.[6] For example, a chest X-ray ordered on an asymptomatic, otherwise healthy fifty-year-old man coming for elective hernia repair reveals a small lesion in the left upper lobe of the lung. This abnormal finding leads to a needle biopsy of the lesion. The needle biopsy results in a collapsed lung and requires a chest tube to reinflate the lung. The pathology analysis of the biopsy is inconclusive. Next, the patient undergoes an open lung biopsy to remove the lesion. This requires three days in the hospital and an additional two to four weeks away from work to recover from the surgery. The pathology results on the biopsy reveal normal scar tissue, which is insignificant. The chest X-ray finding is proven in retrospect to be insignificant. There was no medical indication for the chest X-ray in the first place.

The cost of these unnecessary tests is outrageous. The cost of unnecessary preoperative lab testing in the United States is estimated to be about $1.3 billion per year.[7] You should complain if you suspect your doctor is ordering unnecessary and expensive tests, because many insurance carriers, including Medicare, are often no longer paying for these unnecessary tests.

What You Should Do

In a perfect world, you would be seen in advance of surgery in an anesthesiologist directed preoperative evaluation clinic where you would first undergo a preoperative interview and pertinent physical examination, and only then would the appropriate laboratory tests be ordered based on these findings. This has been shown to be the most cost-effective and efficient medicine[8] and is probably the *best medicine*. This will not always be available to you, so you must be informed and ask questions when appropriate medical practice is not being followed.

First, if you are scheduled for surgery and have not been interviewed or examined by either your regular physician or your surgeon, you should question this oversight. This is the first step required to decide whether *any* preoperative tests are indicated. Batteries of tests are not a substitute for this most important step.

Second, if you are generally healthy, less than seventy years old, have no lung disease, and your physician orders a chest X-ray, you should ask why. A chest X-ray is rarely indicated at any age in the asymptomatic patient, yet they are frequently ordered.

Third, if you are a man less than forty years old or a woman less than fifty years old, are asymptomatic, and your physician orders an ECG, please ask why. There is rarely any indication for an ECG in these patient groups yet they are widely ordered.

Fourth, if you are an asymptomatic male less than sixty years old and your doctor orders any blood tests, please ask why. There is rarely any indication for blood testing in an asymptomatic male under sixty. For a woman less than fifty years old, the only blood tests indicated before surgery are a hematocrit (which indicates the level of red blood cells) and *possibly* a pregnancy test. Women are more likely to have undiagnosed anemia from menses, and thus the blood count is indicated.

Lastly, most asymptomatic pediatric patients over one year old require no laboratory testing at all. If lab tests are ordered on your child that will require a painful needle stick, please ask why.

Conclusion

In today's cattle-drive medical care system, patients are subjected to needless ECGs, chest X-rays, and batteries of blood tests by their physicians in lieu of a proper preoperative history, physical examination, and good medical management. You should be properly evaluated and examined by your doctor before surgery and anesthesia, and you should question unnecessary testing.

4

Why Must I Fast So Long Before Anesthesia?

The ultimate purpose of fasting is to maximize the chances that your stomach will be empty at the time anesthesia begins. Fasting minimizes the chance that undigested food, liquid, stomach acid, and other substances will rise up into your throat and be inhaled into your lungs while you are anesthetized. When you are awake, normal protective airway reflexes will prevent vomit from entering your lungs. When you are in a heavily sedated or unconscious state (e.g., from severe alcohol intoxication, drug overdose, or general anesthesia), you lose those protective airway reflexes, and stomach contents may enter your trachea and lungs unimpeded. If you were to inhale stomach contents into the lungs while anesthetized, you could develop a potentially life-threatening condition called aspiration pneumonia—a pneumonia caused by foreign matter spilling into your lungs.

Aspiration of gastric contents into the lungs can result in a wide range of clinical symptoms, from minor scattered wheezes in the chest to sudden cardiovascular collapse and death depending on the *composition* and *amount* of aspirated material.[1] Acid from the stomach that reaches the lungs causes a chemical burn to the lungs, which may severely impair gas exchange. Large solid particles, like undigested food chunks, cause a different problem. These chunks of matter will physically block small and large airway passages in the lung, and they will prevent effective gas exchange.

When a large volume of material is aspirated, even if it is liquid, it may severely interfere with gas exchange. In its most severe form, aspiration of gastric contents results in sudden respiratory and circulatory failure with severe constriction of the airways. The ability to ventilate the patient and maintain acceptable oxygen levels in the blood may be difficult or impossible.

What You Should Know About Fasting Before Surgery

Anesthesiologists uniformly agree that fasting before elective surgery is an important safety issue and that it is necessary and appropriate. However, there are differences of opinion on how long you should fast prior to surgery to maximize the chances that your stomach will be empty and yet minimize your discomfort from hunger and thirst.

Many studies have been conducted on the time required for the stomach to empty after eating. These studies have generally been done with healthy patients scheduled for elective surgery (patients at high risk for gastric aspiration may require different fasting times and additional interventions to reduce their risk of aspiration).

These studies have shown substantial differences in the rates at which different substances are emptied from the stomach. Stomach emptying depends on many factors, including the type of contents in the stomach (solids versus liquids), the volume of the substance, and the composition of the substance (fat and protein versus sugar and starch).[2] With liquids, the volume ingested is less important than the type of liquid ingested.[3]

Clear liquids: Clear liquids, like water, are emptied from the stomach in one to two hours. Other clear liquids include fruit juices without pulp, carbonated beverages, clear tea, and black coffee. Clear liquids do *not* include alcohol. The American Society of Anesthesiologists (ASA) guidelines for preoperative fasting allow for the patient to consume clear liquids up to two hours preoperatively if they are otherwise healthy.[4] This is a significant advantage for pediatric patients and their families; it minimizes the interruption in the child's daily routine and is a more humane experience for the child and her family. It has the added medical benefit of avoiding the problems of dehydration and hypoglycemia in the infant and small child previously seen with excessively long fasting times.

Full liquids: Full liquids include alcohol and any other liquid not listed as a clear liquid above. Full liquids may take as long as solids to be emptied from the stomach. Depending on the composition of the liquid, it may take six to eight hours to be emptied from the stomach. To be safe, you should refrain from full liquids for a minimum of six hours prior to surgery.

Breast milk: Breast milk is considered to be a special category of liquid. Infants and small children are able to digest breast milk more easily and quickly than nonhuman milk, and it is usually emptied from the stomach within three to four hours. For this reason, infants are allowed human breast milk up to four hours before surgery. However, for nonhuman milk, like formula, a child should fast for a minimum of six hours prior to surgery.

Solid foods: You should fast for a full eight hours or more prior to surgery after consuming a heavy, greasy meal. For a light meal, with minimal grease and protein, you should fast a minimum of six hours prior to surgery to maximize gastric emptying. In Great

Britain, patients are allowed a light breakfast (toast and tea, with no milk added) up to two to four hours prior to surgery. In the United States, where breakfast often consists of greasy bacon, eggs, sausages, waffles, and pancakes, often with maple syrup, the concept of a light breakfast doesn't apply.

What happens when a patient needs emergency surgery after consuming a large meal? With a true emergency, doctors can't wait the desired eight hours for the stomach to empty before surgery. But there are several things that can be done to minimize the risk of aspiration in the patient with a full stomach. First, the anesthesiologist may administer specific medication that can speed emptying of the stomach, or other medications that can neutralize acid in the stomach. Immediately after the induction of general anesthesia, the anesthesiologist will secure the patient's airway by placing a breathing tube in the trachea while a nurse holds pressure on the patient's voice box to prevent stomach contents from rising up into the back of throat. Once the breathing tube is in place, a balloon cuff is inflated to seal the trachea from being contaminated by any food and liquid that may come up while the patient is anesthetized.

Conclusion

An empty stomach at the time of anesthesia induction makes the risk of aspiration pneumonia unlikely. Guidelines for fasting prior to surgery related to the composition of food and drink are given to maximize the chances of an empty stomach. For emergency surgery, it will not always be possible to fast prior to surgery. In these cases, the most important thing you can do is to notify your anesthesia caregiver when you last consumed food and drink and the composition of that food and drink.

5

Should I (or My Child) Receive Sedative Medication Before Surgery?

Anxiety is a normal reaction to anticipated surgery and anesthesia. The vast majority of patients scheduled for surgery will express anxieties about anesthesia. More than half the patients in one study expressed anxiety that they might awake during surgery; others expressed concern about pain after surgery; some were concerned they might not wake up; others feared nausea and vomiting.[1]

Whatever the reasons for your own anxiety, the adverse physiological and psychological consequences of stress and anxiety are well known. Anxiety can activate the fight-or-flight reaction, mediated by the sympathetic nervous system. Activation of the sympathetic nervous system results in adrenaline secretion by the adrenal glands, increased heart rate, increased blood pressure, increased anxiety, and often a sense of doom.

In the healthy adult or child, this reaction may not be life threatening, but it can be quite unpleasant, and there *are* consequences stemming from untreated anxiety. More than half the children who receive general anesthesia and surgery displayed "negative behaviors" for up to two weeks following the procedure.[2] Negative behaviors reported were nightmares, separation anxiety, eating problems, increased fear of doctors, aggressive behavior, bed-wetting, and temper tantrums. In 20 percent of the children studied, these negative behaviors persisted up to six months; in 7 percent they were still evident at a year.[3]

The approach to the patient with anxiety must be individualized to patient's needs. There is no single method or drug to treat anxiety in all patients. Anxiety about anesthesia and surgery isn't always the patient's main concern. If the most important concern of the patient is pain, he should receive a pain medication. If the primary concern is the need to speak with a family member, then he may need a telephone. If the patient desires to confess his sins before the surgery, then he may need to see a priest. The point is that your specific problems, concerns, and fears must be addressed preoperatively.

The Importance of the Preoperative Visit to Reduce Anxiety

There is no doubt that a well-conducted preoperative visit by the anesthesiologist can significantly reduce your level of anxiety.[4] The meeting between you and the anesthesiologist is important for many medical reasons, but it is also an important time to answer any questions about the anesthetic management and to provide psychological support and reassurance. A well-conducted preoperative visit may decrease your postoperative narcotic requirements and shorten your length of stay in the hospital.[5]

Pharmacological Methods to Reduce Anxiety

Once the preop visit is completed and your concerns and questions have been addressed, you may still have significant anxiety.

Administering an anxiety-reducing drug may reduce or eliminate this anxiety. By far and away the most commonly prescribed drug for reducing preoperative anxiety is Versed (midazolam).

Versed is highly effective in reducing preoperative anxiety in both the adult and the child. It is a member of the benzodiazepine family of drugs, the same family of drugs as Valium (diazepam) and Ativan (lorazepam). Versed is about three times as potent as Valium, and it doesn't burn upon injection like Valium. Versed has a considerably faster onset of action than Valium and causes profound amnesia shortly after intravenous administration. The duration of action of Versed is considerably shorter than Valium, which makes it an excellent choice for outpatient surgery.

Outpatient Surgery and Premedication

A spirited discussion often ensues when anesthesiologists discuss premedication for the patient having an outpatient procedure. A few studies report that discharge times in outpatient facilities were prolonged following administration of Versed. Other studies have reported no difference in discharge times with the administration of commonly used doses of Versed. Whether any difference in discharge times exists is debatable, and if there are differences, they are quite small and clinically insignificant. If you are still anxious after the preoperative visit with your anesthesiologist and desire a medication to reduce anxiety, there is no reason you should not receive Versed.

Children and Premedication

The preoperative visit between the anesthesiologist and the child having anesthesia is just as important as the preoperative visit with an adult. Proper psychological preparation of both the parent(s) and the child before surgery is critical. A reassuring meeting between the child, the parent(s), and the anesthesiologist is important; the use of play therapy to introduce the child to the anesthesia experience that is about to occur in age-appropriate ways can also be very helpful.

Pharmacological Methods to Reduce Anxiety in the Child

Despite a good preoperative visit between the child, the parent(s), and the anesthesiologist, and despite age-appropriate explanations to the child about the experience of anesthesia and surgery, the child—like the adult—will often have persistent anxiety. Even the very calm and brave child may have some degree of "meltdown" upon leaving for the operating room. In fact, the silent child and the child that appears aloof and calm during the preoperative visit may be more prone to emotional outbursts upon induction of anesthesia. Many of these children will benefit from sedative medication before the trip to the operating room.

Versed is by far the most widely used medication to reduce anxiety in children before surgery because of its rapid onset, reliability, brief duration of action, and minimal side effects. Children who receive Versed premedication demonstrate significantly less anxiety upon separation from parents to go to the operating room, upon arrival to the operating room, and with the introduction of the facemask to go to sleep than children who did not receive premedication with Versed.

The benefits of Versed premedication for children may extend into the period after surgery as well. In one study, children who received Versed premedication demonstrated significantly fewer negative behaviors (e.g., nightmares, separation anxiety, eating disturbances, excessive fear of doctors) in quantity and quality in the first week following surgery than those children who did not receive Versed premedication.[6] Interestingly, studies have also shown that anxiety levels in the *parents* of pediatric patients are reduced when the child receives Versed premedication.

The route of administration of Versed is often different in the child than in the adult. Adults invariably have an intravenous in place so we can conveniently administer the Versed by this route. Children under the age of ten are generally terrified of needles, so every effort is made to spare them the further anxiety and pain of the intravenous placement until after they have fallen asleep with a mask. For this reason, we often administer Versed to the child either by mouth (oral) or by nose (intranasal).

Intranasal administration: The nasal route of administration is often chosen for the child less than three years old. The onset of sedative effect is rapid by this route—usually less than ten minutes. Some children will be upset with nose drops because they can cause some minimal stinging, so the oral route may be chosen instead.

Oral route: Versed comes in a cherry-flavored syrup that is well received by most children. The dose has to be increased slightly to achieve the same effect as the intranasal route, and it will takes a few minutes longer to work, but effectiveness on the child (and the parent) is similar to the intranasal route.

Should You Accompany Your Child Into the Operating Room for Induction of Anesthesia?

This is a controversial topic that leads to anxiety in parents, children, and anesthesiologists alike. The answer is a definite "maybe." Sometimes a support person will be a calming influence on the child, but at other times they cause chaos.[7]

The first priority is always to consider what is best for the child. Allowing parents or other relatives into the operating room during induction may not always be a calming influence on the child. Parents who are anxious and insistent on being present on induction of anesthesia may transfer this anxiety to their child and will thereby increase the child's anxiety. Some parents have a hard time relinquishing control and care of their child to a stranger, which may create stress for all involved during induction of anesthesia. Some parents are critical of the child or give excessive commands—or even excessive reassurances—and this may increase the child's anxiety.

If a parent plans to accompany his child to the operating room, most facilities require that she be evaluated in advance of surgery to be certain that her presence during induction will benefit the child. It is important to note that even if the parent plans to be present at her child's induction of anesthesia, Versed may still be of benefit to both parent and child. Versed premedication has been shown to provide additional anxiety reduction in the child even when the parent is present at induction.[8] *In fact, a study comparing Versed premedication with a parent present at induction of anesthesia found that Versed premedication was superior to parental presence at induction in reducing the child's anxiety.*[9] Parental anxiety scores are also significantly lower when the child receives premedicated with Versed.

Conclusion

Anxiety is common in the period before surgery. A good preoperative visit with the anesthesiologist can reduce or even eliminate this anxiety. For those patients with residual anxiety after this meeting, especially children, premedication with Versed can eliminate this anxiety and minimize its negative physical and emotional effects.

6

Do I Need an Anesthesia Specialist for My Child?

More than 3 million children receive anesthesia in operating rooms in the United States each year. Countless others will receive anesthesia for diagnostic or painful procedures outside the operating room. Studies of anesthesia related morbidity and mortality during the past fifty years have consistently reported that infants and young children are at significantly greater risk of a serious complication or death associated with anesthesia than the older child or adult. Why?

Infants and small children have striking physiological differences that place them at much higher risk of anesthesia than the older child or adult. Infants and small children have substantially higher metabolic rates and oxygen demand. The infant has much smaller lung volumes, a smaller airway that is more prone to obstruction, and far less respiratory reserve. The infant airway is not only smaller but also anatomically different. The epiglottis is relatively large and floppy; minor airway irritation or infection (croup, epiglottitis) may result in swelling that can cause dangerous narrowing or even closure of the airway. Infants are prone to cold stress, which may lead to cardiovascular instability, decreased oxygen levels in the blood, and bleeding disorders. The physiological conditions present in the infant and small child make them far more prone to life-threatening complications, including hypoxemia (low oxygen level in the bloodstream) and cardiac arrest.[1]

Anesthesia for infants and small children requires specialized equipment and a special skill set. General anesthesiologists are appropriately concerned when asked to anesthetize infants and small children. General anesthesiologists typically receive little specialized training in anesthesia for infants and children; and even if they have received some training during residency, many haven't administered anesthesia to an infant in months or years. The general anesthesiologist is aware that infants and small children are prone to sudden and dramatic airway and cardiovascular deterioration that may be life-threatening. The margin for error in pediatric anesthesia is far less than the older child and adult. If problems are not handled quickly and adroitly, the patient may suffer cardiac arrest and death.

Pediatric Surgery and the Importance of Location, Location, Location

In most industries, there is a demonstrable improvement in efficiency with experience (the so-called learning curve). As a team gains experience, the number of errors decreases, efficiency increases, and the cost of producing an item decreases. This is a quality observed in virtually all human endeavors, not just in industry. Thus operating room conditions are safest and smoothest when everyone on the team is regularly participating in the care of infants and young children.

To properly care for the infant and young child requires appropriately trained and qualified surgical staff, nursing staff, and anesthesia staff in a facility where this type of patient is routinely cared for. Studies show that the "occasional" pediatric surgeon has substantially higher complication rates, including death, than the surgeon who regularly performs surgery on children.[2] It has been shown that surgeons who perform procedures on children as simple as a hernia repair have higher complication rates than surgeons who are specialists in pediatric surgery.[3] There are also differences in mortality between institutions that specialize in pediatric care and hospitals that do not specialize in pediatric patients even for procedures as common as a tonsillectomy.[4]

Conclusion

What the anesthesiologist, surgeon, and hospital do on a regular basis is probably what they do best. I personally would choose an anesthesiologist who is regularly anesthetizing infants and children for my child for *any* surgical procedure being done. I would insist on a surgeon who is a pediatric specialist to perform the surgery. I would allow the procedure to be done only at a facility that regularly cares for infants and children. The added risk may be sufficiently great for your infant or child that you may be willing to travel a greater distance to receive specialized care at a hospital or ambulatory facility that has anesthesiologists and surgeons who are also pediatric specialists.

If your managed-care health plan sends your child for surgery to a facility that is ill-equipped to care for infants and children, that is staffed by individuals who are not adequately trained in the care of pediatric patients, and employs surgeons and anesthesiologists who are only occasionally taking care of pediatric patients—all for financial reasons—please inform the health plan that the scientific literature suggests that this may not be the best medical care for your child and they may be placing your child at added risk.

7

Do I Need an Anesthesia Specialist for My Heart Surgery?

Cardiac surgery is the most invasive and perhaps the most risky of all operations. To accomplish heart surgery, you may be subjected to incredible physiological derangements, like induced cardiac arrest, and placement on a heart-lung bypass machine. In addition, the patient scheduled for cardiac surgery is often sicker and will not tolerate ordinary anesthesia techniques due to severe heart disease and diminished cardiac function. These patients require special anesthesia techniques and monitoring to minimize the risk of the procedure.

The safe anesthesia management for cardiac surgery patients requires special skills and special knowledge that the general anesthesiologist does not often need or possess. To monitor your response to the unnatural manipulations of cardiac surgery and heart-lung bypass and to guide therapy, the cardiac anesthesiologist is required to use high-tech and invasive monitors. These monitors may be placed directly in the heart (the Swan-Ganz monitor) or in the esophagus (transesophageal echocardiography) by your anesthesiologist to monitor heart function and to provide critical information for precise management during and after surgery. In many cases, the surgeon will make decisions about the operation based on the information obtained by the anesthesiologist from these monitors. Highly specialized skills that the general anesthesiologist often does not need or possess are required to safely and correctly insert these important invasive monitoring devices and to correctly interpret the information they provide. It is no surprise that studies have confirmed that the skill and experience of the anesthesiologist have a significant impact on complication rates and outcomes in cardiac surgery.[1] Anesthesiologists who regularly administer anesthesia for cardiac surgery often do it better and safer than those who do not.

Heart surgery requires excellent communication and working relationships between all members of the heart team. Because there are so many steps in heart surgery, and because even a small error can have serious consequences, heart surgery, more than others, requires meticulous standardization of procedures to avoid errors. These factors indicate the need for the heart team to work together regularly to be highly proficient and minimize errors. It is no surprise that studies have consistently demonstrated that complication rates are lower and outcomes are better in hospitals that perform 200 or more open-heart operations per year.[2] The risk to you may be substantially higher if you have your heart surgery performed in a hospital that does fewer than this number.

Conclusion

What the anesthesiologist, surgeon, and hospital do on a regular basis is probably what they do best. If I were scheduled for heart surgery, I would choose an anesthesiologist who is regularly performing anesthesia for cardiac surgery. I personally would have heart surgery only at a facility that is doing 200 or more open-heart operations per year. It may be worth the inconvenience of traveling farther for the improved care.

If your managed-care insurance company sends you for heart surgery at a facility that does substantially fewer than 200 open-heart operations per year for financial reasons, please advise your insurer that the scientific literature suggests that surgical results may be substantially better when performed at a facility doing more than 200 open-heart operations per year. The insurer's choice may be placing you at increased risk.

8

Do My Coexisting Medical Problems Affect the Risk of Anesthesia?

Patients coming to surgery with coexisting medical problems are frequently concerned about how these will influence their risk of anesthesia. Coexisting medical problems may influence risk of anesthesia and surgery, but estimating the risks is a complex issue that depends on many factors, including coexisting medical problems, the contemplated surgery, the anesthesia, and a variety of other variables, many of them unquantifiable (see Chapter 19).

Anesthesiologists use a simple scoring system known as the American Society of Anesthesiologists physical status score to estimate the severity of the patient's preoperative medical conditions. This allows anesthesiologists and researchers to be able to compare the overall health of patients with widely different diseases largely for statistical purposes and research.[1] Patients are assigned an ASA physical status score from 1 to 6 based on their diseases (see Table 8.1).

The ASA physical status score is a grading of your general health coming to surgery and is not dependent on the type of surgery, your age, or your gender. The ASA physical status score is the

TABLE 8.1   The ASA Physical Status Scoring System

ASA Score	Physical Status
ASA 1	A normal, healthy patient.
ASA 2	A patient with mild to moderate systemic disease.
ASA 3	A patient with severe systemic disease that is not incapacitating.
ASA 4	A patient with incapacitating illness that is a constant threat to life.
ASA 5	A moribund patient who is not expected to survive for twenty-four hours with or without surgery.
ASA 6	Organ donor. Brain dead patient for organ harvesting. Included in the physical status scoring system is the designation "E" for emergency.

SOURCE: American Society of Anesthesiologists

overall measure of one important variable in the risk equation: your coexisting diseases coming to surgery. Although the ASA physical status score is *not* a measure of your operative risk, it has been shown to correlate with complications and death associated with anesthesia and surgery.[2] Patients with a physical status score of 3 or greater may have a severalfold higher incidence of complications during and after surgery when compared to ASA 1 and ASA 2 patients. Indeed, in most studies, the number-one factor correlating with complications or mortality associated with surgery was an ASA physical status score of 3 or greater.

When we add "E" (for *emergency*) onto the physical status score, we go from the frying pan into the fire. Numerous studies on risk associated with anesthesia and surgery have identified E designation

TABLE 8.2. **Estimated Risk of Hospital Mortality in Relation to Age, Preoperative Disease, and Surgery**

Preoperative Disease and Surgery		Hospital Mortality		
		Age <50 years old	Age 50-69 years old	Age >70 years old
Chronic heart failure	Elective	0.1%	0.4%	0.8%
	Emergency	0.5%	2%	4%
Renal failure	Elective	0.2%	0.9%	2%
	Emergency	1%	2%	9%
Abdominal surgery	Elective	0.3%	1%	3%
	Emergency	2%	6%	12%
Chronic heart failure and Renal failure	Elective	0.7%	3%	6%
	Emergency	3%	13%	24%
Chronic heart failure and Abdominal surgery	Elective	0.9%	4%	7%
	Emergency	4%	17%	30%
Renal failure and Abdominal surgery	Elective	2%	2%	16%
	Emergency	8%	32%	50%
Chronic heart failure and Renal failure and Abdominal surgery	Elective	6%	22%	37%
	Emergency	26%	60%	76%

SOURCE: Pederson, T., et al. (1990), "A Prospective Study of Mortality Associated with Anaesthesia and Surgery: Risk Indicators of Mortality in Hospital," *Acta Anaesthesiologica Scandinavica* 34: 176–182.

as being associated with a severalfold increase in risk. Emergency surgery on the patient with a physical status score of ASA 3 or higher can be associated with prohibitive risk (see Table 8.2).

What You Should Do

It is clear that as the number and severity of your coexisting diseases increase, then your risk will also increase for any given anesthesia and surgery. You may not be able to change your medical problems before surgery, but you can certainly take steps to reduce your risk of surgery and anesthesia.

If your surgery is totally elective and of dubious value—and there are countless surgeries in this category—I urge you to consider not having surgery at all unless it will clearly improve your quality of life. If you decide to proceed with surgery, there are three areas you should focus your attention to reduce your risk: your health; the anesthesia caregiver; and the location where the surgery will be done.

Your Health

The most important factor is optimizing your health. Do not accept a battery of tests ordered by your doctor as a substitute for a physical examination and real medical care. You want to make sure that you are in the best possible medical condition prior to surgery. If you have high blood pressure, diabetes, heart disease, or lung disease, make sure these are well controlled prior to surgery. If you have chronic diseases and your symptoms are suggestive of worsening condition, have these conditions addressed by your doctor well in advance of surgery. If you feel these conditions are not being well managed, cancel any elective surgery until they are. *Less severe manifestations of chronic disease are associated with marked reductions in risk.*

But there are additional things you must do to improve your general health coming for surgery. If you smoke, stop immediately.

If you do not partake in daily physical activity, do so immediately. If you drink too much, cut down or stop. If you have an unhealthy diet, immediately change it to a healthy one. I recommend these changes to all patients whether they are having surgery or not because they improve quality of life; these changes may also reduce risk of complications associated with anesthesia and surgery.

The Anesthesia Caregiver

Choose the anesthesia caregiver wisely. Many of those who administer anesthesia outside the hospital setting have had little, if any, formal anesthesia training. Many of these "posers" are unable to recognize and treat problems associated with the administration of potent anesthetic drugs. If you are a patient with significant coexisting medical problems and are going to have a procedure requiring the administration of anesthesia, I recommend that you use only a trained anesthesia specialist. If you have complex medical problems, then you are already at increased risk of surgery and anesthesia. Why would you increase your risk even further by having an amateur administer your anesthesia? Go with the expert.

Location, Location, Location

A patient with complex medical problems should have anesthesia and surgery only at a facility that adheres to accepted standards of patient care and accepted standards of patient monitoring and has the appropriate facilities to respond to any adverse event that may occur during or after your surgery. This notion of location is extremely important. The patient with complex disease is more likely to have a problem, and so the facility where surgery and anesthesia are performed must be prepared to promptly respond to any adverse events that may occur. The potential problems with unaccredited facilities and office-based surgery suites are legion. Please read the chapter on office-based anesthesia (Chapter 28) to find out how you can evaluate the quality and safety of an office-based surgery facility.

Conclusion

The nature and severity of your coexisting diseases are perhaps the most important factors influencing your risk of anesthesia. The most important thing you can do, with the help of your doctors, is to be in the best possible medical condition coming to surgery. The more severe your medical problems and the more complex your surgery, the more important this is. Do not accept a battery of tests as a substitute for appropriate management of your medical conditions.

9

Am I at Increased Risk If a Relative Died While Under Anesthesia?

Most people are not at increased risk even though a family member may have died while under anesthesia. However, there are rare inherited conditions that manifest only when the patient is exposed to certain anesthetic agents that may place a related family member at substantially higher risk if the anesthesiologist isn't prepared for the condition or if they do not know the proper anesthetic management or treatment indicated for the condition.

The three most common causes of death under anesthesia for *any* patient, in order of frequency, are: the patient's coexisting medical or surgical diseases that brought him or her to surgery; surgical misadventure; and anesthetic mishap. None of these causes of death will affect surviving family members' risk of anesthesia. These causes of death associated with anesthesia and surgery are by far the most common, and they numerically dwarf all others. But how does the anesthesiologist distinguish between these much more common causes of death associated with anesthesia and surgery and the rare, life-threatening, genetic conditions that manifest only with exposure to certain anesthetic agents?

When Anesthesiologists Become Detectives

When a patient gives the history of a family member dying under anesthesia, the anesthesiologist should attempt to get a clear history of the circumstances surrounding that death to establish the most likely cause of death. Old records documenting the anesthetic and what happened would be helpful, but unfortunately we often find that the relative had surgery thirty years ago in a hospital that no longer exists.

If old charts and reliable information about the relative's death under anesthesia are lacking, the anesthesiologist should try to estimate the contribution of coexisting diseases to the death. It is incumbent on your anesthesiologist to try to obtain this information from old records or from you during the preoperative interview. If the anesthesiologist cannot reasonably attribute your relative's death under anesthesia to underlying disease, surgery misadventure, or anesthesia mishap, then there is small chance that the blood relative's death may be related to a genetically transmitted condition that may potentially affect all surviving family members.

Most genetically transmitted conditions have clinical manifestations that make them readily detectable—hemophilia, muscular dystrophy, dwarfism—and so on. When genetic conditions are known in advance, the anesthesiologist can prepare and administer an anesthetic appropriate to the condition. Unfortunately, certain genetic conditions have no clinical manifestations except when the patient is exposed to certain anesthetic agents.

Malignant Hyperthermia Syndrome

In 1960, a case report appeared in a prominent medical journal describing a twenty-one-year-old man scheduled for surgery who reported to his anesthesiologist that ten of his blood relatives had died during or shortly after the administration of general anesthesia.[1] All the deceased relatives had developed high fevers during or after general anesthesia that preceded shock, convulsions, and death. It was the landmark case description of a rare, inherited disorder that later became known as malignant hyperthermia syndrome.

Malignant hyperthermia (MH) is a disorder of muscle metabolism. The malignant hyperthermia reaction, triggered by certain anesthetic agents, results in an abnormal release of calcium in the muscle cells that results in involuntary, sustained muscle contraction. The sustained muscle contraction results in massive energy expenditure and a hypermetabolic state that is associated with dramatic heat and carbon dioxide production.

Malignant hyperthermia is a genetically transmitted condition. Those patients related to an MH-susceptible person should be treated as if they were MH-susceptible as well. There are differences in gene pools of MH-susceptible individuals. In the Midwest, there are more MH-susceptible families than in other parts of the country. There is a substantially higher incidence of malignant hyperthermia reaction in children and young adults than older patients. The incidence of a full-blown MH reaction is in the ballpark of 1:50,000 anesthetics administered to adults and about 1:15,000 anesthetics administered to children.[2]

The MH-susceptible individual may have the reaction when exposed to certain anesthetic agents called *triggering agents*. Triggering agents are exactly as they sound—they may trigger the reaction. Triggering agents include Anectine (succinylcholine) and all potent anesthesia gases (especially halothane) except nitrous oxide. MH-susceptible individuals will not always manifest an overt reaction even when exposed to known triggering agents. *Indeed, 50 percent of those patients who manifest an MH reaction under anesthesia have had a prior anesthetic without any problem.* Susceptible patients may manifest a reaction at any time during the case. It has even been reported to occur hours after the case was over. One of the very earliest signs of a reaction may be muscle rigidity when the muscle relaxant succinylcholine is administered. Succinylcholine normally causes flaccid paralysis of all voluntary muscles within seconds. When a patient's muscles become diffusely rigid instead of flaccidly paralyzed after the administration of succinylcholine, there is a high probability the patient has MH susceptibility and should be treated accordingly (see below). An unexplained rise in heart rate despite adequate levels of anesthesia is another warning sign of a reaction. Associated with this heart-rate increase is a steady increase in the patient's carbon dioxide production, indicating increased metabolism associated with the uncontrolled muscle contraction.

The dramatic rise in body temperature—the trademark that gave this syndrome its name—can be alarming. The patient's body temperature may rise one degree every five minutes. Malignant hyperthermia syndrome has been described as being cooked from the inside out. If not rapidly and aggressively treated, the malignant hyperthermia reaction will cause muscle destruction, severe metabolic derangement, kidney failure, brain injury, and eventually cardiac arrest and death. Untreated malignant hyperthermia syndrome has a mortality of 70 percent or greater. For successful treatment, early diagnosis and treatment is key.

Diagnosis

There is no diagnostic test (blood test, X-ray, CAT scan, MRI) that will identify the MH-susceptible person in advance. There are only three ways to diagnose the MH-susceptible patient; family history suggestive of MH; when the patient manifests a full-blown MH reaction under anesthesia; and muscle biopsy analysis.

For the majority of the MH-susceptible patients, the first indication they are susceptible is when they have a full-blown reaction under anesthesia. A family history of myopathy (muscle disorder) or prior problem under anesthesia is only present in 30 percent of the patients who are MH-susceptible. Stated in another way, 70 percent of patients who are MH-susceptible have no family history of problems with anesthesia and no family history of myopathy. Any muscle disorder places the patient at higher risk for a reaction. King Denborough syndrome, central core disease, and possibly muscular dystrophy may be associated with MH susceptibility (although available evidence suggests that muscular dystrophy is probably not related to MH).

The only specific diagnostic test for MH susceptibility requires a piece of the patient's muscle tissue (a piece about the size of an adult thumb is required) for analysis. The muscle specimen, usually removed from the thigh of the patient suspected of having MH, is sent to a special laboratory that measures the contraction characteristics of the muscle when exposed to halothane vapor, a known triggering agent. This is called the *halothane contracture test*. The halothane contracture test will identify 90 percent of patients who are MH-susceptible. This test is not helpful in making the diagnosis during the acute MH reaction because it takes several days to obtain the results. We need a very high index of suspicion of MH susceptibility before we are justified in subjecting a patient to the muscle biopsy.

Conclusion

First, if you have *any* family history of unusual reactions to anesthesia (not nausea and vomiting or being "slow to wake up"), you must notify your surgeon as soon as you are scheduled for surgery, and she should arrange for a patient consultation with an anesthesiologist well in advance of surgery. Often, this consultation can occur on the telephone. In this way, the anesthesiologist can identify in advance any special precautions that may need to be taken for your safety.

Second, the malignant hyperthermia reaction can usually be avoided by using special anesthesia techniques if it is known in advance that you have the condition. Even if you do manifest a full-blown malignant hyperthermia reaction under anesthesia, treatment is almost 100 percent successful *if you are being cared for at a facility that has the proper resources and medications to treat this reaction and treatment begins immediately.*

Lastly, if you do have a family history of problems with anesthesia, please be sure you have a trained anesthesia specialist taking care of you at a facility where they have the resources to properly handle a crisis should it develop. Mortality from malignant hyperthermia today approaches zero when you have an anesthesia specialist caring for you at a facility that has the proper resources to handle this crisis and the antidote drug for malignant hyperthermia (Dantrolene).

10

Is it Dangerous to Have Multiple Anesthetics in a Short Period of Time?

It is not at all uncommon for adult and pediatric patients to receive multiple anesthetics in a short period of time for diagnostic and therapeutic procedures. For example, it is not uncommon for a woman to undergo several anesthetics in rapid succession associated with the diagnosis and treatment of breast cancer. There is the initial anesthetic for a breast biopsy. If the initial breast biopsy is positive for cancer, the second anesthetic might be administered for a lumpectomy with limited axillary lymph node dissection. If lymph nodes were positive for cancer cells, the woman might have yet a third anesthetic for a procedure to put in a long-term intravenous access port buried beneath the skin on the chest wall for the administration of chemotherapy.

The administration of multiple anesthetics in a short period is even more common in children. At the Children's Hospital where I work, in a single month we have administered a dozen or more anesthetics to children requiring painful diagnostic or therapeutic procedures.

Your particular risk associated with each anesthetic and surgical procedure will depend on a complex interaction of factors, including your disease, the surgery, and the anesthesia. Generally, the risk associated with multiple anesthetics is simply the additive risk associated with each procedure. Usually, there is no special risk associated with having multiple anesthetics in a short period of time. However, there is an unusual circumstance where patients who are otherwise in good health and undergoing low-risk surgery may have a rare and sometimes devastating reaction to general anesthesia, especially if they have multiple exposures to certain anesthesia gases within a relatively short period.

Halothane Hepatitis

Halothane is an anesthetic vapor that was released for use as a general anesthetic in 1956. Laboratory studies on rats prior to its release showed that halothane was partially metabolized by the liver, but extensive testing suggested there were no adverse effects on the liver. The concern about liver toxicity was related to the use of chloroform as a general anesthetic vapor. Chloroform was known for its wicked dose-related liver toxicity in humans. After extensive studies on rats before its release for use on humans, halothane *seemed* immune from this hazard.

But in 1963, sporadic case reports in the anesthesia literature of unexplained massive liver damage following exposure to halothane caused concern within the anesthesia community.[1] These cases of severe liver damage were seen after relatively minor surgery in healthy patients after having what seemed to be uneventful anesthesia. Because of these reports and the possibility that halothane was more toxic than previously thought, a study (the National Halothane Study) was undertaken to resolve the question.[2] Charts of more than 850,000 anesthetics delivered between 1959 and 1962 were reviewed with the purpose of determining if cases of severe liver injury were caused by halothane or related to the multitude of other factors known to cause liver damage and hepatitis.

The National Halothane Study concluded that although massive liver damage following halothane exposure can occur, it is exceedingly rare.[3] The risk of this complication is greater with multiple exposures to halothane vapor and in the patient with obesity. Fatal liver damage following exposure to halothane was calculated to be approximately one in 35,000 anesthetics.[4] In fact, the number of patients who suffered nonanesthesia-related liver damage following surgery far exceeded the number of patients who had reportedly suffered liver damage from halothane vapor. Halothane hepatitis was found to be an extraordinarily rare occurrence in children. The conclusion of the study was that *unexplained fever and jaundice associated with halothane use might reasonably be considered a contraindication to its subsequent use.*

Conclusion

If you undergoing multiple anesthetics, some of the newer anesthetic vapors are better choices than halothane. Forane has largely replaced halothane as the anesthetic gas of choice for adults. Forane has been available since the 1980s, undergoes minimal metabolism in the liver, and has not been shown in any well-conducted study to cause liver damage directly related to any effect of the vapor. Sevoflurane (Ultane) is replacing halothane as the anesthetic agent of choice in pediatrics. In many hospitals, however, the high cost of Sevoflurane makes halothane the only anesthetic vapor available for pediatric anesthesia.

The most significant risk of any anesthetic is related to the condition of the patient coming to surgery, not the number of anesthetics they have received. Your biggest risk factor for repeat anesthetics is not the anesthetic vapor; it is the reason you need to have multiple surgeries or procedures in a short period of time in the first place. A well-managed anesthetic is far more important than the particular anesthetic vapor used.

11

Will the Anesthesiologist Be Present and Watching Me Throughout Surgery?

If you are curious about this issue, you are actually asking two questions. The first refers to the continuous physical presence by the anesthesia caregiver during your procedure. The second refers to whether the anesthesiologist will be watching you while physically present in the operating room. Both issues are important for the safe administration of anesthesia.

Vigilance is the ability to remain alertly watchful especially to avoid danger. It is also the motto on the seal of the American Society of Anesthesiologists.

The importance of the anesthesiologist as your primary monitor during anesthesia cannot be overstated. No instrument or electronic monitor can take the place of an alert, vigilant anesthesia caregiver. For the first 100 years of the practice of anesthesia, the primary method of monitoring the patient was the astute observation by the anesthesia caregiver. The anesthesia caregiver would observe the depth and frequency of the patient's respiration to assess ventilation, skin color to assess blood flow and oxygenation, and pulse for rate and strength to assess heart function. The key to safety during anesthesia was sustained vigilance of the anesthesia care giver. It still is!

Every single monitor we use in the operating room today requires the interpretative skill of a human. By themselves, monitors do nothing but warn of the status of certain physiological variables of the patient. These physiological monitors are essential, but without a skilled person interpreting the monitors and deciding on the appropriate response, they are useless.

During my anesthesiology residency at the University of California–Los Angeles Medical Center, it was an absolute requirement that a qualified anesthesia caregiver would continuously attend the patient under anesthesia. To do otherwise would have been grounds for immediate termination. When patients would ask me, usually with a nervous laugh, if I would be in the operating room during the entire surgery, I assumed they were kidding, or had some unrealistic fantasy about what happens while they are under general anesthesia. I found out later that it was I who had the unrealistic fantasies about what was occurring in operating rooms around the world!

In 1986, a study on mishaps attributable to general anesthesia that had resulted in serious injury or death to the patient reported that 3 percent of these accidents had occurred while the anesthetist was out of the operating room.[1] In these cases, the accidents were judged to be preventable if the anesthesia caregiver had been in continuous attendance and paying attention during the surgical procedure.

The American Society of Anesthesiologists has standards of monitoring that are recommended for all patients receiving anesthesia. The standards recommended by the ASA are the "gold standard" by which the conduct of the anesthesia caregiver is judged. Monitoring Standard I states categorically that *qualified anesthesia personnel shall be present in the operating room throughout the conduct of all general anesthetics, regional anesthetics, and monitored anesthesia care.*[2] This standard seems superfluous because it is so basic for patient safety. Changes in the patient's status during surgery and anesthesia occur literally in a heartbeat, and this is predictably unpredictable. Those responsible for the patient must be physically present to monitor the patient and quickly detect these changes and respond appropriately.

The practice of leaving an anesthetized patient unattended in the operating room still occurs with regularity. It sounds crazy, but otherwise competent anesthesiologists will regularly drop out of the operating room, sit in the doctor's lounge drinking coffee or conversing on the telephone while a patient under their care is asleep and having surgery. This runs completely counter to ASA monitoring standards, and it is profoundly irresponsible, unethical, and dangerous. It is an egregious violation of standards of patient care. If any patient were damaged as a result of the anesthesiologist leaving her unattended during an anesthetic, it may qualify as criminal negligence.

No anesthesia caregiver can defend the practice of leaving a patient unattended during anesthesia if the patient suffers harm, but how about the more insidious and more common situation of the anesthesia caregiver being physically present in the room but not paying attention to the patient?

There is no doubt that anesthesia morbidity and mortality would be reduced with increased vigilance by anesthesia caregivers. Virtually all studies on mishaps occurring during anesthesia, including death, report that human error is responsible for the majority of untoward events.[3] Of these errors, many are related to lapses in vigilance—failing to detect a problem that was evident and correct it before the patient was harmed.

Vigilance by the anesthesiologist is the best protection that the patient will suffer no harm. Vigilance means the anesthesiologist is continually scanning the surgical field, the anesthesia machine, and all the monitors attached to the patient the way a pilot scans the instrument panel in front of her. This means watching for subtle clues or trends that may be an early warning that something is going wrong or that the patient is not doing well.

Vigilance means the anesthesiologist will detect potential problems early before they become disasters and will respond to them appropriately. A minor problem that goes undetected and uncorrected may have catastrophic consequences. A disconnect between the patient and the anesthesia machine for just a few minutes will likely result in brain damage or death from lack of oxygen. An interruption between the patient and the anesthesia machine is a *potential* disaster. It becomes an *actual* disaster if it goes uncorrected for just a few minutes.

Boredom, Distraction, Fatigue, and Vigilance

The three most common factors associated with decreased anesthesiologist vigilance during a case are boredom, distraction, and fatigue.[4] There are periods during a case when not much is happening, and these are times of potentially decreased vigilance as a result of boredom. Sometimes, anesthesiologists will combat boredom by calling in a competent anesthesia colleague to watch over the patient while they take a short coffee break to sharpen up. Leaving the patient anesthetized and unattended is completely unacceptable, but having one competent anesthesiologist relieve another for a short break is considered acceptable and safe practice. A study conducted on this practice suggests that there is no harm to you, and, in fact, it is likely to improve the vigilance of the primary anesthesiologist.[5]

Other anesthesia caregivers will participate in activities to combat boredom that distract attention away from you. Distractions are a threat to vigilance and contribute to human error. Some distractions in the operating room are unavoidable, but most are completely avoidable. Activities that may distract anesthesiologists include: reading a book, extended conversations on the telephone (most often about matters completely unrelated to your care or medical issues), completing crossword puzzles, listening to talk radio with headphones, paying bills, browsing the Internet with a laptop computer, and, rarely, watching a DVD movie. This list is by no means exhaustive. Some anesthesiologists report that these activities decrease boredom. This is true, but there are abundant studies that show distractions from any cause will create an environment prone to accidents and errors, and some of those errors will be catastrophic.

Anesthesia is accurately compared to flying an airplane. There are many similarities between airline pilots and anesthesiologists. Commercial airline pilots do not participate in distracting activities while flying the aircraft. No sane passenger would fly on an airplane if he believed the pilot would be engaged in these kinds of activities during the flight.

Another common factor reducing anesthesiologist vigilance is fatigue. Extreme fatigue can severely degrade human performance and the ability to concentrate on a task. Several cases of physician fatigue leading to critical judgment errors and patient harm have achieved national media coverage. In one case, an anesthesiologist was allegedly asleep during a case while the child under his anesthesia care died on the operating table. Studies have shown that the motor skills, judgment, and mental performance of a person who has been up for twenty-four straight hours is the equivalent of a person who is legally drunk.[6]

Conclusion

A moment or two of distraction from the patient during anesthesia isn't likely to cause catastrophe, but the anesthesiologist's sustained attention to anything other than the patient may represent a general cavalier attitude toward vigilance and monitoring that may in fact endanger the patient. Eventually, behaviors that distract the anesthesia caregiver from watching the patient will lead to preventable mishaps. Although it will never be possible to completely eliminate human error from any human endeavor, decreased vigilance caused by distraction may increase the probability that errors will occur and, when they do occur, will result in decreased detection of those errors. Any attention diverted from the patient during anesthesia should be minimized.

As the patient, your role is to candidly ask the question posed at the outset of this chapter and insist on an honest answer. It is entirely appropriate for you to request that your anesthesia caregiver minimize any activities that will divert his or her attention from you while you are asleep. If you discover your anesthesiologist has been up all night working, it would be entirely appropriate to ask for another anesthesiologist who hasn't.

This candid discussion will likely cause many anesthesia caregivers to reexamine their primary responsibility to watch over you and to reevaluate some of their common practices to combat boredom.

PART II

General Anesthesia

12

What Is General Anesthesia and How Is It Administered?

On Friday, October 16, 1846, at approximately 10:30 in the morning, the first public demonstration of general anesthesia occurred at the Massachusetts General Hospital in Boston. The operation was scheduled to begin at 10 A.M., but the anesthetist, William T. G. Morton, a part-time dentist and full-time flimflam man, was late. He was waiting for the delivery of the glass bottle apparatus invented the day before that he would use for the administration of ether vapor to induce anesthesia. The patient was a housepainter named Edward Gilbert Abbott who was to have a growth removed from the left side of his neck by surgeon J. C. Warren. Warren was one of the founders of the Mass General Hospital and a Dean of the Harvard Medical School.

In front of a gallery of physicians, medical students, and a newspaper reporter, seated in the steep, domed amphitheater, Morton used ether liquid contained inside the specially designed glass bottle with a mouthpiece for the patient, Mr. Abbott, to inhale gaseous ether vapor. After several minutes of inhaling from the mouthpiece, Abbott became unconscious.

Warren performed the surgery for the removal of the mass on the neck in a matter of minutes, without Abbott demonstrating any evidence of pain. Upon the completion of surgery, Warren turned those watching from gallery and said, "Gentlemen—this is no humbug."

Oliver Wendell Holmes, who was a spectator in the amphitheater that morning, wrote, "The state should, I think, be called 'Anaesthesia.'" Holmes is credited with naming this revolutionary process *anaesthesia* from the Greek word meaning "insensible" or "without feeling." Within weeks, much of the civilized world knew of ether and the discovery of surgical anesthesia.[1]

General anesthesia should not be confused with ordinary sleep. When you are in a state of normal sleep and someone slices through your abdominal wall with a razor-sharp scalpel you will not remain asleep. General anesthesia is thus quite different than sleep. General anesthesia might better be described as a reversible, drug-induced coma during which a patient will not perceive or respond to painful stimuli (surgery). The characteristics of an ideal general anesthetic would include unconsciousness, lack of recall of events, absence of muscular response to surgery, diminished or absent response to pain associated with surgery, and *reversibility*. These characteristics can be summarized in the four *A*'s of general anesthesia:

- *Analgesia*—absence of pain
- *Amnesia*—loss of retentive memory
- *Anesthesia*—unconsciousness
- *Akinesia*—absence of motion

How Do General Anesthetic Agents Work?

The numerous complex theories of how general anesthesia agents work may be best summarized in three words: *We don't know.* The various chemicals known to induce the state we call *general anesthesia* are extremely diverse structurally. It is still a mystery how these diverse chemicals result in the state of general anesthesia. It is highly unlikely that these structurally diverse chemicals cause general anesthesia by one single mechanism.

Brain physiologists have tried to elucidate the mechanism by which these diverse chemicals induce an anesthetic state. However, these same brain physiologists are uncertain of the mechanism responsible for the state we call *consciousness*, therefore it is difficult to explain how anesthetic agents cause *unconsciousness*. Some physiologists believe that there are specific locations in the brain that are responsible for consciousness. Other physiologists believe that consciousness is the result of the interaction of many brain areas working together. One theory of anesthesia hypothesizes that anesthetic drugs inhibit certain specific areas of the brain, resulting in unconsciousness. The second theory postulates that unconsciousness is the result of globally depressing brain function with these chemicals. There is one area in which brain physiologists do agree; general anesthesia drugs block transmission of nerve impulses at the *synapse*, where one nerve abuts the next. The specific mechanism by which this inhibition occurs is not understood.

How Is General Anesthesia Administered?

There are many similarities between the different stages of an airplane flight and general anesthesia, and the analogy helps answer this question. The pilot's perspective on a flight may be conveniently divided into four distinct stages: *preflight, takeoff, cruising altitude,* and *landing*. The corresponding four phases of a general anesthetic may be divided into: *preoperative evaluation of the patient* (preflight), *induction of general anesthesia* (takeoff), *maintenance of general anesthesia* (cruising altitude), and *emergence* (landing).

Preflight: Preoperative Evaluation and Preparation of the Patient

Pilots are trained to carefully check their aircraft, the weather, and their flight plans before they ever taxi down the runway. Failure to do so invites disaster. The preflight check will often pick up a potential problem that should be addressed before the aircraft leaves the ground. The anesthesiologist should be similarly thorough in her approach to the patient having anesthesia.

A thorough preoperative evaluation of the patient is important. Knowing the patient's relevant medical history and physical condition is essential to planning a safe anesthetic. If there is something wrong with the aircraft identified in preflight, it must be addressed or corrected before proceeding to takeoff even if it means canceling the flight. So it is with the patient before general anesthesia. If there are conditions in the patient that should be optimized before surgery, or questions that need to be answered, the takeoff should be postponed or cancelled until the questions are answered and the conditions are corrected.

A pilot and crew are compulsive about checking the aircraft before a flight to be certain everything is in proper working order so there are no surprises on takeoff or once in the air. Likewise, the vigilant anesthesiologist must be certain all her equipment is prepared and in good working order in advance of takeoff. An essential part of this preflight check is a methodical inspection of the anesthesia machine to make sure it is functioning properly. Between 5 percent and 20 percent of anesthesia mishaps are related to equipment failure.[2] Most of these equipment failures could have been detected in advance of surgery and avoided if the anesthesiologist had done a thorough check of the anesthesia machine and other required equipment before anesthesia was started.[3]

The modern anesthesia machine is a self-contained anesthesia gas delivery system, a carbon dioxide absorbing device, a mechanical ventilator, and possesses a variety of safety features and multiple backup systems to detect malfunctions in gas delivery, oxygen delivery, and ventilation (see Figure 12.1).

The modern anesthesia machine can deliver up to three different anesthetic gases using specific *vaporizers*. A vaporizer is a cylindrical container the size of a small thermos that is filled with liquid anesthetic agent. This liquid is converted to a vapor and delivered into the gas mixture traveling from the machine to the patient. The anesthesia machine additionally delivers oxygen and nitrous oxide.

The modern machine has many redundant safety features that are designed to prevent patient harm. Sensors detect if inadequate amounts of oxygen are being delivered to the patient; other sensors detect excessively high or excessively low pressures in the breathing circuit hoses that bring gases from the machine to the patient. These sensors sound an alarm when there is a loss of pressure in the system associated with a disconnection between the patient and the anesthesia machine or when the pressure in the breathing circuit is too high (indicative of obstruction). Another monitor on the machine detects if the amount of ventilation is insufficient. These safety features have markedly reduced catastrophic patient injuries during general anesthesia. But they are not foolproof. They

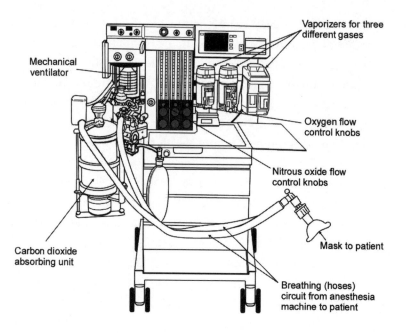

Figure 12.1   The Anesthesia Machine

The anesthesia machine is the self-contained apparatus used to deliver anesthesia gases and oxygen and remove exhaled carbon dioxide gas. Additionally, it has many safety features and a mechanical ventilator.

still require that the person operating the anesthesia machine correctly interprets and responds to the machine's alarms.

The anesthesia machine delivers its gas mixture to the patient via plastic hoses called the breathing circuit (see Figure 12.1). This breathing circuit interfaces with the patient by one of three airway devices: the facemask, the laryngeal mask airway (LMA), or the endotracheal tube (see Chapter 13).

If everything passes inspection in "preflight" with the patient and the equipment, and after all the physiological monitors are applied to the patient, then we are prepared for takeoff (see Chapter 14).

Takeoff: Induction of General Anesthesia

Safely getting the plane into the air without incident requires maximum vigilance. Many things are happening simultaneously; failure to detect a problem and react quickly during this critical time will result in disaster. This is true of the induction of general anesthesia as well.

Induction of general anesthesia takes the patient from a state of wakefulness to deep coma in a matter of seconds using potent anesthetic drugs that may cause severe physiological derangements. Pushing anesthesia medication into the patient's intravenous line at induction is similar to a pilot pushing the throttle of the airplane on takeoff. Once the jet engines are at maximum thrust and the plane achieves 180 knots on the runway, the aircraft is committed to takeoff. Once the anesthesiologist has pushed the medication into the patient's intravenous line to induce general anesthesia, she is committed to the induction.

Induction of anesthesia can be a stressful time for both the patient and the anesthesiologist. Anesthesiologists know that induction of general anesthesia is a time when a disproportionate numbers of accidents occur. Monitors have been attached to healthy anesthesiologists during induction of general anesthesia and have revealed a high incidence of cardiac rhythm abnormalities in the anesthesiologist during this time associated with surges of fight-or-flight hormone release.

There are two methods commonly used to induce general anesthesia. The first method is the use of potent anesthesia gases to induce anesthesia, or *inhalation induction*. When the patient inhales these anesthesia gases, he will be rendered unconscious in a matter of minutes. The second method to induce general anesthesia, *intravenous induction*, is accomplished by injecting potent anesthesia agents directly into the bloodstream using the patient's intravenous line.

Anesthesia By the Inhalation of Anesthesia Gases

Historically, general anesthesia was first induced by inhalation of ether vapor in 1846. Ether vapor was soon followed by the use of chloroform vapor in England. The use of nitrous oxide gas as a supplement to ether and chloroform vapor came some twenty-five years later with the development of compressed nitrous oxide in a cylinder. Anesthesia by inhalation of these gases was the primary method of anesthesia induction for almost a century after the first use of ether.

Induction of anesthesia by inhalation of anesthetic gases is still a very popular method of inducing anesthesia for children who often have a severe fear of needles. The child inhales the mixture of anesthetic gases coming from the anesthesia machine by facemask until unconscious. With modern anesthetic gases, this occurs quite rapidly, typically in one to three minutes.

Anesthesia By Intravenous Injection

Most adults find the idea of inhaling anesthetic gases via a facemask objectionable. The preferred method of anesthesia induction in adults is by intravenous injection of the anesthetic drug. Intravenous induction results in a very rapid transition from awake to general anesthesia. This is smoother and swifter than inhalation induction.

Cruising Altitude: Maintenance of General Anesthesia

Most pilots relax a bit when the plane has been brought to cruising altitude without incident and everything seems to be going smoothly. Frequently, pilots will put the plane on autopilot, indicating that a certain stability has been achieved. This is similar to the anesthesiologist when the patient is anesthetized and the maintenance phase of anesthesia has begun. The anesthesiologist must maintain anesthesia for the duration of the surgery. Regardless of whether the patient was induced by inhalation or intravenous methods, the most common technique of maintenance of general anesthesia is by administering a combination of inhalation (gases) and intravenous agents.

At cruising altitude, if the weather is good and there are no engine problems, the pilot can relax until the landing. Unfortunately, the weather may turn bad suddenly, or problems can develop with the airplane engine, and this will require the pilot's utmost attention. Anesthesia is similar. Surgery is often a major physiological trespass, and some patients do not tolerate it well. Many adverse events can occur during the maintenance phase of the anesthetic: bleeding, fluid shifts, cardiac instability, problems with lung gas exchange, and so on. These changes in the patient's condition must be recognized and treated. Vigilance must remain high during the maintenance phase.

Landing: Emergence from General Anesthesia

Landing an airplane is another period of heightened vigilance for the pilot. The flight may have gone perfectly, but if the pilot plants the nose of the plane into the ground at landing, it was all for nothing. The emergence from anesthesia, or waking up at the end of the procedure, is similar to landing the plane. Many critical changes are happening as the patient emerges from his drug-induced coma and must resume his own vital functions, like respiration. Pain medications are added intravenously to alleviate surgical pain as the patient rapidly breathes off the anesthesia gases. The patient must have acceptable vital signs, an adequate breathing pattern, and adequate levels of consciousness before they are ready to be transported from the operating room to the recovery room.

In the recovery room, for the first time since the induction of general anesthesia, the anesthesiologist will transfer the care of the patient to the specialized nurses in the postanesthesia care unit (see Chapter 21).

Conclusion

General anesthesia takes the patient from wide awake to drug-induced coma in a matter of seconds and maintains this state for the duration of surgery. During the surgery, general anesthesia keeps the patient unconscious, without pain, without memory, and without movement, all the while maintaining the patient's vital functions as close to normal as possible. Within minutes of the termination of general anesthesia, the patient is returned to consciousness to begin the recovery from surgery.

13

Will a Plastic Tube Be in My Windpipe During Anesthesia?

Any discussion of the plastic tube in the windpipe during anesthesia—or *intubation*—generally elicits a visceral response from patients and medical personnel alike. Even many surgeons and nurses have misconceptions about the plastic tube that anesthesiologists place in the trachea (the endotracheal tube). Patients are often concerned about the prospect of having this plastic tube inserted in their trachea and the discomfort this may cause. But it's important to know—indeed, it is now legally required—for the anesthesiologist to discuss why this tube may be used unless you, with knowledge, decline to hear about it.

What Is the Purpose of the Endotracheal Tube?

The purpose of the endotracheal tube is to provide you with a safe and secure airway during surgery and general anesthesia and, in some cases, to control your ventilation after surgery. There are other devices and methods that may be used to establish and secure

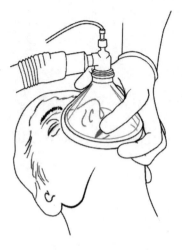

Figure 13.1   The Facemask

Anesthesia gases can be administered by the anesthesia face-mask, which snugly fits around the patient's nose and mouth.

your airway as well. The three most common methods used to control your airway during anesthesia are: the facemask (see Figure 13.1), the laryngeal mask airway (Figure 13.2), and the endotracheal tube (Figure 13.3). All three methods are commonly used, but there are specific reasons and indications why the anesthesiologist may choose one airway device over another.

The Facemask

Before the facemask was developed in 1917, anesthesia was administered by a rag soaked in ether stuffed in a glass bottle with a mouthpiece for the patient to inhale gaseous ether vapor. The *poor man's anesthetic* was just a rag soaked in ether applied over the patient's face. The facemask was revolutionary for its day. With an airtight seal

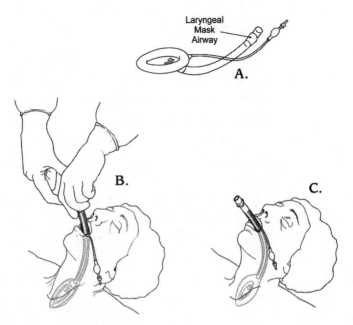

Figure 13.2   The Laryngeal Mask Airway

A. The laryngeal mask airway.

B. Inserting the laryngeal mask airway.

C. The final resting position of the laryngeal mask
   airway above the vocal cords.

around the mouth and nose, the facemask is a method to deliver anesthesia gases and oxygen from the anesthesia machine via the breathing circuit to the patient. The patient will breathe the anesthesia gases efficiently in the mask (see Figure 13.1). The administration of anesthesia by facemask is still widely employed for very brief procedures where the anesthesiologist has direct access to the patient's airway or for the inhalation induction by a mask.

The Laryngeal Mask Airway

The laryngeal mask airway is another device commonly used to secure the patient's airway. The LMA is made of soft rubber and is inserted via the mouth into the back of the throat and rests above the vocal cords after you are asleep (see Figure 13.2). The end of the LMA coming out the mouth is connected to the anesthesia breathing circuit. For many surgeries, your airway can easily and safely be managed with the LMA. Because the LMA does not enter the trachea or pass through the vocal cords, it is less irritating to the airway and throat than the endotracheal tube.

The LMA is not a sufficiently secure airway for all cases or completely free of side effects. The LMA can still cause a sore throat; the LMA does not protect against aspiration pneumonia the way a cuffed endotracheal tube can. Ventilation cannot be controlled as precisely or as reliably with the LMA as can be done with the endotracheal tube. Although it is a revolutionary airway device that is quite useful, the LMA has not replaced the need for the endotracheal tube.

The Endotracheal Tube

In 1920, rubber tubes designed to deliver inhaled anesthetic gases directly into the trachea were introduced into anesthesia practice. These tubes were called "endotracheal tubes" to denote their position within the trachea. The introduction of endotracheal tubes was a major advance in anesthesia that allowed for controlled mechanical ventilation and more invasive surgery. Today this tube is made of soft plastic and is inserted either through the mouth or the nose through the vocal cords into the trachea (see Figure 13.3). The end of the endotracheal tube coming out of the mouth is connected to the anesthesia breathing circuit where anesthesia gases and oxygen

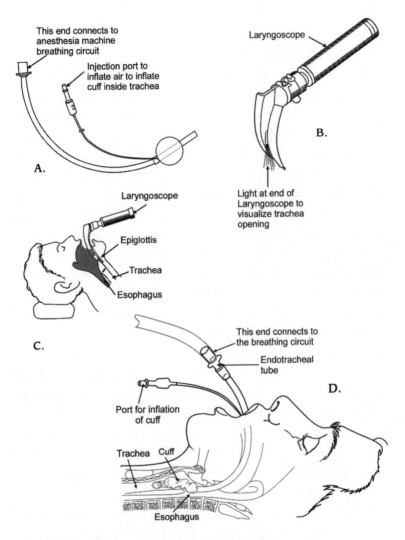

Figure 13.3   The Endotracheal Tube and Laryngoscope

A. The endotracheal tube—cuff inflated.
B. The laryngoscope is a device used by the anesthesiologist to
   illuminate and visualize the vocal cords through which the
   endotracheal tube will pass.
C. The use of the laryngoscope in the anesthetized patient.
D. The endotracheal tube inside the trachea.

are delivered to the patient. A low-pressure cuff (or balloon) on the outer portion of the endotracheal tube is positioned inside the trachea and is inflated to form an airtight seal between the endotracheal tube and the trachea (see Figure 13.3 A). This airtight seal prevents any stomach contents, fluids, or secretions from entering into the trachea or the lungs during anesthesia. Inhalation of gastric contents into the lungs (aspiration pneumonia) can have dire consequences (see Chapter 4). The use of cuffed endotracheal tubes has dramatically reduced the incidence of this complication.

The endotracheal tube is usually placed in the trachea after you are asleep and removed before you are awake. The process of inserting the endotracheal tube into the trachea is called *intubation*. A laryngoscope (see Figure 13.3 B) is a device used to visualize the vocal cords through which the endotracheal tube will be passed. The laryngoscope blade used to visualize your vocal cords is essentially a steel tongue depressor with a tiny light bulb at the end of it. The laryngoscope blade is placed in your mouth *after* you are anesthetized and used to sweep your tongue out of the way and to shine light on the vocal cords so the anesthesiologist can see the opening to the trachea (Figure 13.3 C).

The vast majority of patients are unaware an endotracheal tube was used unless they experience a mild sore throat. In some major surgeries, like open-heart surgery, this tube may be left in place following surgery and the patient mechanically ventilated for several hours. If you require an endotracheal tube after surgery, you will usually receive sedative medication to keep you comfortable until it is removed.

When Is Endotracheal Intubation Necessary?

There are a variety of reasons that the anesthesiologist may choose to use the endotracheal tube during surgery. One of the most important reasons to use an endotracheal tube is to protect your lungs from aspiration pneumonia. When the endotracheal tube is in the trachea with the cuff up, aspiration pneumonia is exceedingly unlikely. Patients at high risk of aspiration (e.g., morbid obesity, pregnancy, hiatal hernia, bowel obstruction, etc.) may require an endotracheal tube even for brief procedures.

If your surgery requires the use of mechanical ventilation and the use of muscle-paralyzing agents, an endotracheal tube is probably safest. If the surgery requires that your anesthesiologist is some distance from your airway (e.g., head and neck surgery), then the use of an endotracheal tube is probably safest. Major surgery invading a body cavity (chest, abdomen, brain) is safest with an endotracheal tube. Surgeries that are long are probably more safely managed with an endotracheal tube. An endotracheal tube is required for any patient who will require mechanical ventilation postoperatively.

Complications Associated with Endotracheal Intubation

Most often there are *no complications* associated with the placement and use of an endotracheal tube. Sometimes during insertion of the endotracheal tube, you may have minor trauma to your lip (fat lip) or teeth (chipped tooth). If you have preexisting dental disease, unusual airway anatomy, or you bite down hard while the endotracheal tube is in place, you could suffer more extensive dental damage, such as a dislodged tooth. Sore throat is probably the most common complaint. Typically, this is mild and resolves itself within twelve to twenty-four hours without any therapy. Vocal-cord damage is very uncommon, and if it does occur, it usually resolves spontaneously over a matter of days or weeks. The endotracheal tube can be an airway irritant to you if you have significant lung disease (asthma, chronic bronchitis, or emphysema), but this is usually easily managed.

In about two or three out of every 1,000 patients, the endotracheal tube can be quite difficult to insert. If you have ever had an anesthesiologist tell you that she had difficulty inserting the endotracheal tube in you, you should speak with your anesthesiologist and warn her of this fact. With modern monitoring devices and high-tech airway equipment, even the most difficult intubation can be handled safely, but it will require extra preparation and equipment for this.

Conclusion

As unpleasant as the mental images might be, the use of the endotracheal tube is routine and markedly increases the safety of general anesthetic in cases where it is indicated. The complications associated with its use, when they do occur, are usually minor.

14

How Will I Be Monitored While I'm Under Anesthesia?

On October 16, 1846, William Morton administered sulfuric ether vapor to Gilbert Abbott at the Mass General Hospital for the removal of a neck tumor in the first public display of surgical anesthesia. The only monitor attached to the patient was Morton himself. For more than a century and a half since Morton's first public demonstration of ether, the anesthesia caregiver remains the single most important monitor assigned to the patient—*but this alone is not enough.*

The Purpose of Monitoring

The purpose of monitoring in anesthesia is to provide early warning that something is wrong and to allow adequate time to detect and correct the problem. One of the primary functions of the anesthesiologist is to maintain your body's vital functions as close to normal as possible during anesthesia and surgery. Through the use of advanced monitoring devices, the anesthesiologist can detect changes that may warn of developing problems and then use these monitors to guide interventions and therapies to restore your body's vital functions to as close to normal as possible. Since the 1980s, minimum standards of anesthesia monitoring were codified and adopted by the American Society of Anesthesiologists.[1] Knowing what these standards are will help you understand the anesthesiologist's responsibilities and additionally will help you understand the purpose of the various monitors that will be attached to you during your surgery.

The ASA Standards of Intraoperative Monitoring

> Standard I: Qualified Anesthesia Personnel Shall Be Present in the Room Throughout the Conduct of All General Anesthetics, Regional Anesthetics, and Monitored Anesthesia Care[2]

The Ultimate Monitor

Monitors are only as good as the person using them. The anesthesiologist's primary function is your safety during anesthesia and surgery and to maintain your body's vital functions as close to normal as possible. Adverse, life-threatening events can occur suddenly and without warning during all types of anesthesia. These life-threatening problems often require rapid intervention to avert disaster. To fulfill this responsibility, the anesthesiologist must be present and vigilant at all times.

The anesthesiologist must integrate the information gathered by his/her senses and the physiological monitoring tools and act upon this information to keep you safe. Monitors give numbers; they need to be interpreted and evaluated according to a clinical picture or information available. The anesthesiologist is the only monitor that can evaluate, interpret, synthesize, and react appropriately to this information for the safety of the patient.

> Standard II: During All Anesthetics, the Patient's Oxygenation, Ventilation, Circulation, and Temperature Shall Be Continually Evaluated

Monitoring Oxygen in the Patient

Just twenty years ago in the operating room, the oxygen level in the patient's blood was estimated by observing the color of the fingernails and lips. If the patient's lips and nail beds were pink, the oxygen level was assumed to be adequate; if they were blue, the oxygen level was determined to be inadequate. This was, of course, an extremely crude and unreliable method for detecting inadequate oxygen levels in the patient.

Today we can continuously and accurately monitor oxygen in the patient's blood by using a device called a *pulse oximeter*. The pulse oximeter (or *oxygen saturation monitor*) utilizes the fact that oxygenated arterial blood absorbs light at one wavelength (bright red) and that venous blood that has already delivered its oxygen to the tissues absorbs light at a different wavelength (dark red). Using a light-sensor probe on a finger, an ear lobe, or even the nose, the color of red is analyzed and the device determines the oxygen level in the patient's blood continuously. The pulse oximeter has an audible pulse tone that parallels the measured oxygen level in the blood. If the measured oxygen level is adequate, the device has a high-pitched sound with each heart beat. As oxygen levels in the patient fall, the pitch falls in proportion to the decrease in oxygen saturation.

The pulse oximeter allows for early detection of even subtle problems with oxygenation long before they would have been detected using visual methods or arterial blood gas analysis. Twenty years ago, the first detection of inadequate oxygenation in the patient under anesthesia might be a cardiac arrest. Today, even minor drops in oxygen levels of the anesthetized patient can be immediately detected and corrected by the anesthesiologist using the pulse oximeter.

Monitoring Ventilation

Inadequate ventilation (i.e., breathing) has been identified as one of the most important factors associated with brain damage and death in the anesthetized patient. A patient who is anesthetized and paralyzed is completely dependent on the anesthesiologist for breathing. Even a brief interruption in ventilation could lead to catastrophic brain damage or death. Consequently, there are multiple monitoring devices that are used by the anesthesiologist to detect and warn of inadequate ventilation in the patient before it leads to disaster. Two of the most important methods for continuously measuring the adequacy of the patient's ventilation are the pulse oximeter (discussed above) and the *expired carbon dioxide monitor.*

A quantum leap in patient safety during anesthesia occurred with the introduction of a monitor that was able to continuously measure expired carbon dioxide gas. As oxygen is consumed in the metabolic processes in the body, carbon dioxide gas is produced. Carbon dioxide gas is transported from the tissues of the body dissolved in the bloodstream to the lungs, where it is eliminated during respiration. The measurement of carbon dioxide gas expired by the patient is the most direct measure of the adequacy of the ventilation.

Continuous monitoring of carbon dioxide during general anesthesia gives your anesthesiologist a great deal of important information other than just adequacy of your ventilation. The presence of carbon dioxide confirms that the breathing tube used during anesthesia is in the correct position in the trachea. If the carbon dioxide suddenly disappears during surgery, this indicates a potentially serious problem (e.g., a disconnect between the patient and the breathing circuit, a kinked breathing tube, a dislodged breathing tube, a plugged or obstructed breathing tube, and various other life-threatening problems that must be attended to promptly by the anesthesiologist).

Monitoring Circulation

Both anesthesia and surgery may cause marked elevations and reductions in blood pressure suddenly and without warning; continuous monitoring of the patient's cardiovascular status is essential. Blood pressure, pulse, and electrocardiogram monitoring are used to assess overall cardiovascular function in the anesthetized patient.

Monitoring Blood Pressure

Automated blood pressure monitoring devices used in the operating room today can accurately measure the patient's blood pressure as often as necessary, typically at one- to three-minute intervals. The machine automatically inflates the cuff at predetermined time intervals; even if the anesthesiologist is distracted, the blood pressure is still measured. If your blood pressure falls outside narrow limits—either too high or too low—the monitor will alarm and alert the anesthesiologist. Modern automated blood pressure monitoring devices are highly reliable, even in tiny infants.

Monitoring the Electrocardiogram

Continuous ECG monitoring of the anesthetized patient didn't routinely occur until the late 1950s. Since then, ECG monitoring devices have become quite sophisticated, not only for detecting heart rate and rhythm disturbances but also for detecting inadequate blood supply to the heart (ischemia). The continuous ECG monitoring allows detection and treatment of episodes of coronary insufficiency before they progress into a heart attack.

Temperature

It is important to detect changes in the patient's temperature for other than the briefest surgery. Your temperature may drop during surgery from a variety of potential sources: a cold operating room, an exposed patient being prepped with cleaning solutions that are at room temperature; cold fluids administered via the intravenous; and so on. It is important to monitor the patient's temperature and to detect changes in temperature and correct it. Your anesthesiologist will monitor your temperature using a tiny, disposable, plastic-coated wire placed in the mouth or attached to the skin during anesthesia.

Monitoring Depth of Anesthesia

Currently, there are no accepted standards for monitoring the patient's level of consciousness during anesthesia. This is an interesting paradox. Anesthesiology is a discipline with the primary purpose of administering drugs to render a patient unconscious for surgery and yet has developed no standards or recommendations for monitoring the patient's level of consciousness during anesthesia.

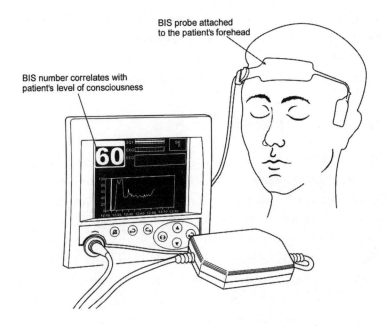

Figure 14.1   The BIS Monitor

The BIS monitor measures brain electrical activity in the anesthetized patient to determine the depth of unconsciousness.

Currently, there is only one Food and Drug Administration–approved depth of anesthesia monitor, called the BIS monitor (see Figure 14.1).

The BIS monitor is a device that is technically simple to use and interpret, provides information about the patient's level of consciousness, and guides the rational administration of anesthetic agents to the patient's level of consciousness. A sticky, flat plastic strip about the size of a large Band-Aid is applied to the patient's forehead and around to the right temple (see Figure 14.1). This probe is connected to a monitor that measures electrical signals from your brain, interprets brain-wave activity, and displays a number that correlates with level of consciousness. The BIS monitor, or some level-of-consciousness monitor like it, will become a standard of care for patient monitoring during anesthesia in the future.

Monitoring Muscular Paralysis

If a muscle-paralyzing drug is used to facilitate surgery and anesthesia, the anesthesiologist will use an electronic device to accurately monitor the extent of your muscle weakness using a device called a *nerve stimulator*. This device guides the administration of muscle relaxant drug to avoid excessive or prolonged weakness. The nerve stimulator is often attached to your wrist and, using an electrical pulse stimulator, the twitch of your thumb is measured and will indicate the level of muscle paralysis. At the end of the case, this monitor will guide the anesthesiologist in the administration of medications to reverse your muscle paralysis if needed.

Exceptional Monitoring

The anesthesiologist may need more invasive monitoring in addition to the standard monitoring mentioned above if you have a severe coexisting disease or if the surgery is especially extensive or invasive—like heart surgery. Special catheters about the diameter of a spaghetti noodle may be placed into the heart via a large vein in the neck to monitor heart function during certain surgeries. In addition, during major surgeries, the anesthesiologist may insert a special catheter about the size of a small intravenous line into an artery in your wrist to directly measure blood pressure. These monitors are more costly and more invasive than standard monitoring devices, but for certain operations they are required to guide your anesthesia and surgical management. These monitors are sufficiently out of the ordinary that the anesthesiologist should discuss the need for these monitors with you in detail before surgery.

Conclusion

Adherence to accepted standards of monitoring in anesthesia have contributed to the dramatic improvement in the safety of anesthesia and the reduction in catastrophic injuries to the anesthetized patient. A substantial body of evidence suggests that the marked decrease in serious injuries associated with anesthesia is in part related to the use of the patient monitoring devices discussed above.[3]

15

Will I Be Paralyzed During Anesthesia?

One of the essential characteristics of general anesthesia is *akinesia*, or lack of patient movement. The development and use of muscle relaxant drugs without any anesthetic properties to specifically produce akinesia in order to facilitate surgery during general anesthesia was a major advance in the field of anesthesiology. Though patients understand the need for immobility during surgery, they are still terrified of the prospect of being paralyzed and awake during surgery. The truth is that your anesthesiologist *will* often use a muscle-paralyzing drug during anesthesia to facilitate surgery and avoid the dangers associated with deep levels of general anesthesia.

The term *muscle relaxant* used in this discussion does *not* refer to drugs in the Valium family. The muscle relaxant drugs employed in anesthesia are relatives of *curare*, the plant extract used by the Amazon Indians on the tips of arrows and darts to paralyze big game, including *Homo sapiens*. In fact, the first muscle relaxant to be introduced into clinical anesthesiology was curare in 1942.[1] This was the seminal event that marked the beginning of the widespread use (and occasional abuse) of muscle relaxant drugs in the specialty of anesthesiology. Muscle relaxants (more correctly, *neuromuscular blocking drugs*) are an important supplement to many general anesthetics.

Why Muscle-Relaxant Drugs Are Used

Prior to the use of muscle-relaxant drugs, the only method available to the anesthesiologist to assure the patient would not move during surgery was by the administration of very deep levels of ether anesthesia. As anesthesia was deepened with ether, the patient's muscles would relax, but this relaxation came at a heavy price to the patient: Deep ether anesthesia would produce dangerous levels of cardiac and respiratory depression. Cardiovascular collapse and respiratory arrest with ether anesthesia were not uncommon before the introduction of curare. With the availability of muscle-relaxant drugs today, the anesthesiologist does not have to subject you to dangerously deep levels of general anesthesia to achieve akinesia and adequate muscle relaxation for surgery.

How Do Muscle Relaxants Work?

Muscle relaxant drugs attach to specific sites at the junction between certain nerves and the muscles they innervate. Once the muscle relaxant drug binds at this site, it prevents the nerve transmission from reaching the muscle; thus the muscle is incapable of contracting. Muscle paralysis caused by these drugs may be terminated either by waiting until the effects of the muscle-paralyzing drug wear off spontaneously, or, if necessary, the anesthesiologist may administer specific drugs that will completely reverse the muscle paralysis in a matter of seconds.

Which Muscles Do the Muscle Relaxants Work On?

Muscle-relaxant drugs work only on your voluntary muscles. If muscle-relaxant drugs worked on all types of muscles in the body, then your heart would stop, because the heart is also a muscle. That doesn't happen. The muscle relaxant will paralyze any muscle that you can move voluntarily, including your diaphragm. Patients who have received muscle-relaxant drugs cannot breathe adequately by themselves, which is why the anesthesiologist must assist or control your breathing.

Clinical Uses of Muscle Relaxants

There are many reasons why the anesthesiologist may use muscle relaxants during anesthesia. The most common use for muscle-relaxant drugs is to facilitate the insertion of the endotracheal tube. Operations within the abdomen are also greatly facilitated by the use of muscle-relaxant drugs. It is difficult for the surgeon to achieve adequate exposure of the organs inside the abdomen without dangerously deep levels of anesthesia unless muscle-relaxant drugs are used. Any surgery where patient movement might result in disaster may also be an indication for the use of a muscle relaxant.

Monitoring Paralysis

The anesthesiologist should always monitor your response to muscle-relaxant drugs if they are used. They can do this with an electronic device called the *nerve stimulator*. The nerve stimulator is applied to the skin over a nerve, usually at the wrist, and a series of electrical impulses are delivered. The electrical stimulation of the nerve causes the muscle it supplies to contract. Based on the magnitude and characteristics of the muscle contraction, the anesthesiologist can precisely determine your level of muscle paralysis; this information will guide the administration of muscle-relaxant drugs during your surgery, and at the end of surgery your anesthesiologist can use this device to determine if you require the administration of drugs that can reverse any residual paralysis you might have.

Conclusion

The introduction of curare-like drugs into anesthesia practice was a tremendous advance. Muscle-relaxant drugs provided excellent surgical conditions in lighter planes of anesthesia than previously possible. The use of muscle-relaxant drugs is a valuable addition to anesthesia, but their inappropriate use without providing adequate levels of anesthesia may result in patients who are awake and paralyzed during surgery. This phenomenon, called *awareness*, is the subject of Chapter 16.

16

Is It Possible to Be Awake During Surgery?

More than half of all patients coming for surgery express anxiety that they might be awake during surgery.[1] The very idea of being awake during one's own surgery conjures up images of horror stories by Edgar Allen Poe. The technical term for this nightmare is called *awareness*. That is, you are *aware* of what is happening during surgery when the anesthesiologist and surgeon think you are anesthetized.

Awareness means that you were conscious of what occurred during some or all of your surgery when you were supposed to be unconscious. You were awake when you were supposed to be asleep. What often adds to the terror of the situation is that the patient with awareness has often been paralyzed with a muscle-relaxant drug, rendering him unable to communicate through movement or speech of this predicament to anyone else in the room. Although rare, this can happen.

Types of Awareness

There are two types of awareness. *Awareness with recall* is where you were aware of what was happening during your surgery and afterward were able to tell us (i.e., recall) what you experienced. The second type of awareness is a little trickier and generally ignored. *Awareness without recall* is where you were aware of what was happening during your surgery but are unable to recall this experience afterward. It's like the age-old question: *If a tree falls in the forest and no one is there, did it make a sound?* In this case, if you were awake during surgery but can't recall it afterward, did it really happen? The answer is an *unequivocal yes*. It can happen, and it does happen. How often this happens no one knows.

The Inappropriate Use of Muscle Relaxants

In the early 1950s, fascinated with muscle-relaxant drugs, anesthetists in the United Kingdom popularized a technique of anesthesia consisting of nitrous oxide, oxygen, and curare along with small doses of narcotic. This technique became known as the *Liverpool technique* after its place of origin. The goal of the Liverpool technique was to avoid deep level anesthesia and to have the patient wake up very quickly at the end of surgery. Unfortunately, this regimen of ultralight anesthesia was often inadequate for surgery. If the patient moved during surgery, the anesthetist using the Liverpool technique, instead of giving more anesthesia, which is the appropriate response, would give more curare to abolish movement.

Before the introduction of muscle relaxants into clinical anesthesia in 1942, a common problem was that patients were too deeply anesthetized (with the attendant risk of cardiac and respiratory depression). With the introduction of the Liverpool technique and excessive reliance on muscle-paralyzing agents, the opposite problem was observed. Reports in the literature began to appear that described patients who were awake but paralyzed during surgery.

Incidence of Awareness

How frequently does awareness occur? These studies only identify patients who had awareness with recall. The anesthesia literature reports the overall incidence of awareness with recall is somewhere between one in 250 anesthetics and one in 500 anesthetics.[2] If we assume that approximately 15 million general anesthetics are administered in the United States each year, then somewhere between 30,000 and 60,000 patients will have awareness with recall each year in this country.

In situations where anesthesia techniques require large doses of muscle relaxants and low doses of anesthesia gases, the incidence of recall may be substantially higher than the incidence reported above. Reports indicate that up to 1 percent of women undergoing a cesarean section under general anesthesia have awareness with recall during some portion of their surgery.[3] In a study of cardiac surgery patients, more than 1 percent had awareness with recall during some point of their surgery.[4] The incidence of awareness during major trauma surgery may be several times higher than this.[5]

How many patients have awareness without recall? No one knows. The incidence of awareness without recall is difficult, if not impossible, to study prospectively. It would be unethical to conduct a study where patients were intentionally made to be awake during surgery, so we might determine how many of them actually recalled the experience. No sane patient would agree to be a participant in such a study.

Consequences of Awareness

The good news is that the overwhelming majority of patients who have awareness during surgery do not report feeling physical pain—or at least they don't remember feeling pain—during the period of awareness. The literature suggests that only about one in five or one in ten patients who experience awareness will report physical pain.[6] One in four patients describe physical sensations—like tugging, pressure, and touch—during the period of awareness but that these sensations were *not* associated with pain.

There are ramifications of being aware during surgery other than the possibility of physical pain. For many people, this might be considered a traumatic psychological experience. There have been reports in the literature of patients who experienced awareness with recall who have developed subsequent neurosis.[7] The neurosis, similar to posttraumatic stress disorder, is characterized by insomnia, anxiety, depression, irritability, repetitive nightmares, preoccupation with death, and an intense fear of hospitals and doctors.[8] This neurosis may be worsened if the surgeon, the anesthesiologist, or the patient's family or friends try to convince the patient that the experience was imagined.[9]

The potential for psychological trauma caused by awareness is significant and should not be trivialized. The incidence of psychological trauma following awareness may never be known because current data only include awareness with recall. If we assume there are many patients who experience awareness without recall, they too experience the trauma of being aware during surgery, but they do not consciously recall it. These patients may suffer psychological trauma but never understand why. This traumatic experience may influence thought and behavior in ways that we—and they—do not understand. These patients may experience excessive free-floating anxiety, nightmares, depression, irritability, and phobias postoperatively. The consequences of awareness during surgery are not limited to the patient. A number of awareness cases have resulted in medical malpractice claims against the involved anesthesiologist. In a study of anesthesia medical malpractice claims, almost 2 percent of all claims against anesthesiologists are related to patient awareness.[10] The cost of malpractice claims for awareness range from $1,000 to $600,000. The most common complaint in the malpractice action is temporary emotional distress; 10 percent of patients in this study claimed they were suffering from posttraumatic stress disorder.[11]

Preventable Causes of Awareness

Awareness is preventable in many cases, but not all. Prevention of awareness may be accomplished by the anesthesia caregiver thoroughly checking the anesthesia machine prior to starting the case, by vigilance during the case to be certain anesthetic agents are being delivered in sufficient quantities to reasonably predict the patient will be asleep, and by using muscle-relaxant drugs only when indicated and necessary during surgery.

In about one-fourth of the cases of awareness reviewed in one study, the anesthesia caregiver mistakenly administered a muscle-relaxant drug to the patient instead of the intended drug to induce general anesthesia. This is called a *syringe swap* in anesthesia lingo, and it leaves the patient wide awake and paralyzed.

Other simple vigilance errors on the part of the anesthesiologist may result in awareness. For example, if the anesthesia liquid in the vaporizer on the anesthesia machine runs out in the middle of the case and this is not promptly recognized by the anesthesiologist, the patient will soon become conscious. A medical malpractice claim for awareness was settled for more than $100,000 because the anesthesiologist had delivered an anesthetic without realizing the vaporizer was empty. The patient received no anesthetic gas from the vaporizer and was aware during surgery. The patient was given a muscle relaxant, so he was unable to move or otherwise alert the anesthesiologist that he was awake.

Awareness That May Not Be Preventable

There are types of surgery where awareness is more likely to occur through no error on the part of the anesthesiologist. Anesthesia administered in the setting of trauma, shock, or situations of patient instability demand anesthetic techniques that make awareness more likely. In these situations, the patient may be harmed or killed if standard anesthetic doses and techniques are used. In these cases, the number-one priority of the anesthesiologist is the survival of the patient. The incidence of awareness during anesthesia for severe trauma may exceed 10 percent.[12]

There are other types of surgery that, due to the requirements of the situation and through no error on the part of the anesthesiologist, may result in a substantially higher incidence of patient awareness. Cardiac surgery[13] and cesarean section performed under general anesthesia[14] are the two most commonly cited.

When general anesthesia is administered for a cesarean section, consideration must be given to the effects of the anesthesia on the unborn fetus and the excessive bleeding in the mother that may result from administration of even moderate doses of anesthesia gases. The safety of the mother and fetus dictates an anesthetic regimen calling for low concentrations of anesthesia gases.

This is a situation known to be associated with a higher incidence of awareness.

Cardiac surgery patients are another group that are at higher risk for awareness. Many patients scheduled for open-heart surgery have significant cardiac impairment and are not candidates for even moderate doses of anesthetic gases. The use of low doses of anesthetic gases increases the potential for awareness. The second circumstance that places heart surgery patients at higher risk for awareness is the time they spend on the heart-lung machine. Many anesthesiologists give little or no anesthesia gases during this time, which makes this a period where the patient is at higher risk for awareness.

Treating the Patient with Awareness

When an anesthesiologist is informed postoperatively that a patient under her care is reporting that he was awake during surgery, there is a natural tendency toward denial or avoidance. The typical first response is for the anesthesiologist to try to convince the patient, the family, and even the caregivers involved that the patient was only dreaming (perhaps saying, "Dreaming under general anesthesia is normal," which, by the way, is not true). If a patient is in such a light plane of anesthesia that he is able to dream and recall the experience, he was inadequately anesthetized for surgery. If the anesthesiologist is unable to convince the patient he was dreaming or hallucinating, she may try to convince the surgeon, the nursing staff, and even the family members that the whole experience described by the patient is imagined.

The tactics must change if the patient can recount specific events or words spoken in the operating room verbatim that occurred while he was presumed to be asleep. Even the wiliest anesthesiologist must acknowledge the undeniable fact that the patient was awake during at least some of the operation. In this case, many anesthesiologists will enter avoidance mode and avoid a candid discussion with the patient of what occurred.

None of these approaches to the patient who has experienced awareness is recommended. In fact, they are all potentially harmful to the patient. The healthiest approach for both anesthesiologist and patient is for the anesthesiologist to compassionately listen to the patient and, if the claims are genuine, validate the patient's claims that they may have been awake at some time during their surgery. This may lessen the intensity of the neurosis associated with the experience of awareness. It may also help avoid a medical malpractice lawsuit.[15]

A study of medical malpractice claims regarding awareness revealed that much of the patient's distress and anger focused more on the failure of the anesthesiologist to give a proper explanation about the cause of the awareness rather than the awareness itself. Plaintiffs reported that the malpractice suits might have been avoided had the anesthesiologist approached the problem in a straightforward manner, listened to the patient sympathetically, and openly discussed what had happened and why it happened.[16]

Conclusion

First, the chance of you having awareness during surgery is quite low. A review of studies on awareness suggests that the incidence of awareness with recall has decreased dramatically since the 1970s. Studies of awareness between 1960 and 1973 reported rates of awareness four to six times higher than more recent reports.[17] Additionally, the vast majority of patients who have awareness will *not* feel pain.

Second, there is a Food and Drug Administration–approved level-of-consciousness monitor now available for use during anesthesia (the BIS monitor) that indicates your level of consciousness during surgery. With proper use of the BIS monitor, the reported incidence of awareness is substantially lower than that reported in the literature without the use of the BIS.[18] It may be worth asking for, especially in surgeries known to be at high risk for awareness.

Third, if your anesthesiologist appears to be hurrying or in a rush, please ask her to slow down and be careful. Many of the preventable cases of awareness (and other critical errors and accidents as well) are the result of your anesthesiologist, in haste, injecting a muscle-paralyzing drug before the drug to induce general anesthesia ("syringe swap"). Simply avoiding this one error can prevent more than 25 percent of all cases of awareness.

Fourth, ask your anesthesiologist if she has completed a thorough anesthesia machine check as recommended by the American Society of Anesthesiologists. Part of this preflight machine check will detect an empty anesthesia vaporizer that could result in you being aware during surgery.

Finally, if you are one of the rare patients who experiences awareness during your surgery, please bring this to the attention of your surgeon and your anesthesiologist. The most important reason to do this is for your mental health, but it is also important that the anesthesiologist is made "aware" of this situation so that she may explain to you what happened and why.

17

How Does the Anesthesiologist Know How Deeply I'm Asleep During Surgery?

No doubt you want to be asleep during surgery and unaware of what is occurring, but you might also be concerned that you will receive too much anesthesia—more than is required. Obviously, you don't want too much or too little anesthesia; you want just the right amount. How do anesthesiologists monitor your depth of anesthesia to determine how much anesthesia to administer? The truth is, they usually don't; they largely guess.

The only completely reliable measure of *inadequate anesthesia* is patient recall after surgery. The opposite extreme is the patient who complains that she didn't come out of anesthesia for hours or days. The good news is that the number of patients who receive excessive anesthesia far outnumber those who are inadequately anesthetized and experience awareness during surgery. Anesthesiologists will tend to anesthetize patients deeper than is necessary to be certain they will not have awareness or move during surgery. The real question, then, is: How does the anesthesiologist assess your depth of anesthesia to avoid giving too much or too little anesthesia?

Assessing Depth of Anesthesia

More than 150 years after the first public display of surgical anesthesia, most anesthesiologists still *infer* your depth of anesthesia from your physical signs. Anesthesiologists are still taught in their training that physical signs like heart rate, blood pressure, sweating, tearing, and gross movement are *indirect*, or *surrogate*, indicators of the patient's depth of anesthesia. Yet no research has ever shown that these physical signs correlate in any predictable or measurable way with the patient's level of consciousness. In fact, the clinical signs that are widely used by anesthesiologists to assess depth of anesthesia are notoriously inaccurate and unreliable for predicting depth of anesthesia. In a study of patients who had awareness during general anesthesia, only a small number manifested any physical signs of light anesthesia.[1] The anesthesiologist should be monitoring these physical parameters for many reasons, but they are not a reliable indicator of depth of anesthesia.

Most anesthesiologists would consider responses to surgical stimulation like increased heart rate, increased blood pressure, and movement as signs of light anesthesia and would deepen your anesthesia. However, there is no scientific way to correlate these physical signs with your depth of anesthesia. Using these physical signs as an indicator often results in excessive amounts of anesthesia administered to abolish heart-rate and blood-pressure response to surgical stimulation even though you are deeply unconscious. Conversely, a patient undergoing heart surgery may have low blood pressure and a slow heart rate in response to anesthesia even though she is awake and paralyzed during surgery.

Movement is another physical sign commonly used to gauge depth of anesthesia. When a patient moves, she is probably inadequately anesthetized, but if the patient is anesthetized to the point where she does not move, is the patient barely unconscious or in a deep coma? We don't know. Movement doesn't correlate in any scientific way with depth of anesthesia. To abolish all movement in all patients using anesthesia means that many patients will be given excessive amounts of anesthesia.

Dose-Response Curves and Depth of Anesthesia

Anesthesiologists also rely on a detailed knowledge of pharmacology to guesstimate the amount of drug you will require to be fully anesthetized and not move during surgery. *Dose-response curves* are determined in the laboratory on healthy human volunteers and define the dose of the anesthesia drug or gas required to produce unconsciousness and failure to move in response to painful stimuli. In order to assure that you are unconscious and do not move, the anesthesiologist will generally administer substantially more anesthesia drug than is required to be certain you are unconscious and will not move during surgery.

Is it harmful if the anesthesiologist gives you more anesthetic drug than is required? In the usual range of anesthesia excess, the answer is *no*. There is *no* evidence that it is harmful to you other than the possibility of slightly increased incidence of minor side effects like a slower wakeup, increased nausea and vomiting, and increased drowsiness after anesthesia. However, the best practice of all would be the precise administration of anesthesia drugs based on your measured level of consciousness, not based on your blood pressure, heart rate, or movement. Ideally, the anesthesiologist would administer the anesthesia drug based on a direct measurement of your depth of consciousness so that he doesn't give either more or less than necessary.

Directly Monitoring the Patient's Depth of Anesthesia

The technology to directly monitor your level of consciousness under anesthesia already exists. The electroencephalogram (EEG) has been in use for decades by neurologists to measure seizure activity and other pathological brain states through the electrical output of the brain. The EEG is occasionally used in the operating room to measure brain-wave activity for certain specialized surgeries like neurosurgery, but unfortunately the technology is extremely complex and cumbersome. The EEG varies for each different anesthetic agent, making it too complex and distracting for the average anesthesiologist to set up and continuously interpret during the case. Additionally, the standard EEG tracing usually requires the expertise of a neurologist for correct and rapid interpretation. The time and labor involved in applying numerous EEG leads to the patient's head and the size of the EEG monitor also make it impractical to use in the operating room except in extraordinary cases.

The BIS Monitor

The BIS monitor has been developed for use in the operating room to continuously monitor the depth of unconsciousness of the anesthetized patient.[2] The BIS has simplified the complex EEG into a single, averaged signal for easy use and interpretation by any anesthesiologist. A monitoring probe is placed on the patient's head and held by an adhesive strip that can be applied in seconds. The BIS monitor converts your EEG signal, which directly correlates with your level of consciousness into a single number between 0 and 100 that is displayed continuously on a monitor screen (see Figure 14.1). The BIS had been extensively tested on humans who were given a variety of anesthetic agents, and these studies have shown a high degree of correlation between the BIS number displayed and the patient's level of consciousness.[3] The BIS monitor is the only Food and Drug Administration–approved and commercially available monitor to measure level of consciousness under anesthesia. Studies have shown that patients monitored with the BIS receive significantly less anesthesia drug and wake up faster than patients who were not monitored with the BIS.[4]

BIS monitoring does not completely eliminate awareness. However, the incidence of awareness reported in the literature with BIS monitoring was far below the incidence of awareness without BIS monitoring.[5] Interestingly, in several cases of awareness with the use of the BIS, the numeric score displayed on the BIS monitor indicated that there was a high probability that the patient was awake. That is, the BIS monitor warned the anesthesiologist that the patient had a high probability of being conscious. The BIS monitor only warns about the patient's level of consciousness; it does not indicate how the anesthesia caregiver should respond to this information.

The BIS monitor is by no means perfect. However, no monitor used in the operating room is perfect; *under certain conditions* every monitor used in anesthesiology will fail or give inaccurate information. This does not invalidate their importance or make them useless. On the contrary, these monitors are essential in making the process of anesthesia safer and better. The anesthesiologist must be knowledgeable about the shortcomings of the monitor and the conditions under which the information may be inaccurate or misleading.

Conclusion

The methods anesthesiologists generally use to assess your depth of anesthesia, like heart rate, blood pressure, and movement, are quite crude, but these methods invariably result in the administration of more anesthesia drug than you require; therefore, awareness is highly unlikely. The ideal practice of anesthesia, however, is the use of a specific monitor that measures your depth of unconsciousness, like the BIS monitor, to more precisely guide the administration of anesthetic drugs.

18

Does General Anesthesia Have Any Lasting Effects on Mental Function?

In a 1950s report on this subject, more than one-third of close relatives or friends of an elderly person (more than sixty-five years-old) who underwent anesthesia for major surgery reported that the patient "has never been the same" since the operation.[1] In this report, the close family or friends reported the patient had new onset of mental changes, behavioral changes, and/or neurological changes. Some of these changes were reportedly permanent and severe. Does this really happen, or is this just a myth?

Although extremely rare in persons under the age of sixty-five, postoperative mental, behavioral, and neurological impairment in the elderly is quite real, has been well documented, and may be significantly underappreciated. With approximately 35 million Americans over the age of sixty-five and the current life expectancy of American women over eighty, and American men well over seventy, a huge number of patients are at risk for this complication. Fortunately, the vast majority of postoperative mental changes seen in the elderly patient will be temporary.

Short-Term Changes in Mental Function

Short-term changes in mental function are commonly seen after surgery and anesthesia. The most common short-term change in the elderly is *delayed emergence* from anesthesia, which means that the patient is slow to wake up from anesthesia. In the elderly patient, delayed emergence may result from a decreased ability to metabolize or eliminate anesthetic drugs or increased sensitivity to drugs due to age-related changes in organ function. This results in a longer-than-normal duration of anesthetic effects.

Postoperative delirium is another common short-term mental status change seen postoperatively in the elderly. Delirium, by definition, is a *transient* disorder with a sudden onset of mental-status changes characterized by confusion, disorientation, hallucinations, delusions, and overactivity of psychomotor autonomic nervous system function. Patients with delirium have disorganized and incoherent thinking. Short-term memory is impaired. Patients are often disoriented to time, but not infrequently they are also disoriented to place and person. Attention disturbance is always present, with the patient easily distracted. The patient often has no idea where they are, why they are there, and at times do not even recognize family members. This is usually seen on the first or second postoperative day, and symptoms are worse at night. The literature reports between 10 percent and 60 percent of elderly patients may experience postoperative delirium depending on the magnitude of surgery and the age of the patient.

Cognitive impairment is also commonly seen in the elderly patient after surgery and anesthesia and may occur with or without other overt mental status changes. Cognitive impairment includes problems with memory, learning, understanding, and reasoning. These changes may be quite subtle in the absence of other overt mental status changes, sometimes only picked up with sensitive testing.

Long-Term Changes in Mental Function

Persistent cognitive impairments following surgery and anesthesia are not unheard of. Mental changes are still clinically evident in 5–10 percent of elderly patients for weeks or months after surgery.[2] The numbers differ depending on the study reviewed. In one study, clinically evident mental dysfunction persisted for up to six weeks in 5 percent of patients above age seventy.[3] In another study, a significant number of elderly patients still had cognitive deficits at three months.[4] Most of these patients will eventually make a full recovery to their *baseline* function prior to surgery.

Fortunately, permanent neurological deficits following anesthesia are rare. Permanent neurological deficits may be the result of structural brain injury related to stroke, bleeding in the brain, or brain injury from other causes (e.g., lack of oxygen). The exact incidence of new structural brain injuries following surgery are somewhat difficult to determine in the elderly patient because their baseline brain scans are often abnormal, making it difficult to sort out age-related brain changes from new structural lesions.

The Cause

Before anyone rushes to attribute these short-term and long-term mental changes to anesthesia and surgery, it is important to note that elderly patients admitted to the hospital for medical problems have similar or even higher rates of cognitive dysfunction and delirium than elderly patients after anesthesia and surgery! The incidence of delirium in elderly medical patients has been reported to be 25–50 percent depending on the age and degree of illnesses of the elderly patients studied.[5] Mental changes seen in elderly hospitalized patients clearly isn't limited to those who have had anesthesia and surgery. Mental changes are seen with about the same frequency in all hospitalized elderly patients.

Additionally, if these mental-status changes were related to general anesthesia, we would expect that there would be a greater number of patients with postoperative cognitive dysfunction after general anesthesia than after spinal anesthesia. That isn't the case.[6] Studies have generally shown that the incidence of delirium and cognitive dysfunction are the same whether the patient had general anesthesia or spinal anesthesia. This suggests, but does not prove, that the postoperative mental effects aren't related to the anesthesia.

The only factor that has been consistently associated with long-term mental changes following anesthesia and surgery is advanced age. The effects of aging make the elderly more susceptible to the mental changes seen postoperatively. The susceptibility to these changes is related to the condition of the patient's body (biological age) rather than their exact age in years (chronological age). Some elderly persons have the physique of a much younger person and the effects of aging have been slowed; these elderly patients may be less susceptible to postoperative mental changes.

Why Are the Elderly Susceptible to These Mental-Status Changes?

The answer is not known with certainty, but there are several likely reasons. Age-related decline in liver and kidney function results in a decreased ability to metabolize and eliminate drugs, which results in significantly slower elimination and clearance of these drugs from the bloodstream with increased effects—and side effects. The elderly brain is more susceptible to injury and metabolic derangement than the younger brain and less tolerant of it. Alcohol and sedative abuse is common in the elderly, and withdrawal syndrome with delirium may result from sudden cessation of these substances in the hospital. Prevalent psychological factors in the elderly, like depression, dementia, and anxiety, often are associated with postoperative mental decompensation.

Conclusion

If you are more than sixty-five years old and having major surgery requiring hospitalization, there are things you can do to lessen the chance you will have postoperative delirium, and if you do have delirium, to lessen the chance you will have complications from it.

- Optimize all your medical conditions preoperatively. Studies have repeatedly shown that the better your medical conditions are managed before surgery, the better you will do after surgery. Your regular doctor should aggressively treat your high blood pressure, diabetes, and heart and lung conditions prior to surgery. Aggressive medical management before and after surgery is associated with a lower incidence of delirium.[7] Do not accept a battery of tests by your doctor as a substitute for good preoperative medical management of your medical diseases.

- Next, you should ask your regular doctor *in advance* of surgery who will be managing your *medical* problems after surgery during your hospitalization. Surgeons are excellent with surgical problems, wound issues, and so on, but they are not specialists in the management of high blood pressure, heart conditions, lung conditions, and diabetes. If your medical conditions are managed aggressively in the hospital after surgery, this may decrease your chance of mental-status changes after surgery and other complications as well.[8]

- If you are a heavy alcohol or sedative drug user, please honestly inform your anesthesiologist and surgeon of this fact. Sudden cessation of these substances may result in withdrawal symptoms, and often frank psychosis, twenty-four to forty-eight hours later. Your doctor can prescribe medication that will prevent withdrawal from these substances while you are in the hospital and lessen the chance of acute withdrawal syndrome.

- If you have clinical depression or an anxiety disorder, you should have these conditions treated before surgery. Elderly patients with untreated depression or high anxiety levels have a much higher incidence of mental-status changes after surgery compared to those without such conditions.[9]

- Carefully choose where you will have your surgery performed if possible. *Postoperative nursing care is critically important.* You want to be sure that the nurse caring for you will recognize if you are developing mental-status changes and institute appropriate precautions to prevent you from accidentally harming yourself. The delirium you have after surgery will invariably resolve, and you will likely fully recover; however, if you fall out of bed and sustain a skull fracture and bleed into your brain, this may cause permanent injury. This does happen with disturbing regularity, especially in facilities with inadequate nursing staffs. You can inquire with the hospital liaison what the ratio of nurses to patients is on the hospital floor where you will be cared for. An acceptable patient-to-nurse ratio on a normal acuity floor is around five-to-one; in an intensive care unit the ratio should be only two-to-one.

- Lastly, if you are able, have a family member or friend at your bedside while you are in the hospital. This person can provide many benefits, but the most important one is to make sure you are being adequately cared for. Do not underestimate the effect this has on your caregivers; they are well aware that someone else is paying attention to what they do—and don't do—if you, the patient, are unable to act on your own behalf.

19

What Is the Risk of Anesthesia?

Reports of anesthesia-related mishaps and disasters appear in the electronic and print media with disturbing regularity. The public is aware that administration of anesthesia is associated with risk, but they are not clear if death associated with anesthesia is a rare occurrence with marginal practitioners or if this is an unpredictable and unavoidable event even with good practitioners. If you are like most patients, you have contemplated this question before surgery, and like most patients, you hesitated to directly ask your anesthesiologist about the risk associated with anesthesia. Parents of children about to undergo anesthesia are often more concerned about the risk of anesthesia than the risk of surgery. No matter what you may have heard in the media, read in textbooks, or heard at home, *the risk of anesthesia for an individual patient cannot be quantified.*

The Studies on Anesthesia Risk

Since the 1950s, there have been numerous studies published on the risk of anesthesia. Collectively, these studies lack uniformity of study design, they lack uniformity in their methods of data collection, and they lack complete objectivity.[1] Yet published data on the risk of anesthesia are quoted as if they were hard facts. They aren't. They are crude estimates. Although these studies may have flaws and the reported numerical risk of anesthesia varies, this does not mean that they have no value. On the contrary, these studies have been extremely helpful in identifying the factors that influence the risk of anesthesia—and what can be done to make anesthesia safer.

The numerical risk assigned to anesthesia varies widely from study to study, but one clear trend emerges: The risk of anesthesia has declined dramatically during the past half-century. A landmark study on mortality associated with anesthesia in 1954 reported that anesthesia was the primary cause of death in one out of every 2,680 patients.[2] In 1987, in the United Kingdom, a large study on mortality associated with anesthesia reported that only one in 187,000 patients succumbed from anesthesia.[3] In another study, the one reporting the highest anesthesia-related mortality in the 1990s, calculated the overall risk of death attributable to anesthesia at about one in 20,000 operations.[4] Depending on the study cited, the risk associated with anesthesia is between eight and seventy-five times lower than it was in the 1950s.

The reported risk of one in 187,000 in the study cited above is the calculated risk derived from all patients coming to surgery. That is, the sickest patient coming in for heart surgery is included with the conditioned athlete having a hernia repair. I assure you that the risk for the heart surgery patient is significantly greater than one in 187,000, and the risk of anesthesia for the conditioned athlete having hernia repair is probably significantly lower than one in 187,000. *The calculated statistics for the risk of anesthesia do not apply to individual patients.*

Studies of risk associated with anesthesia have looked at different groups of patients to clarify the differences in risk. The risk of anesthesia to the healthy patient is not the same as the risk to the morbidly ill patient. A study of more than 1 million healthy patients (ASA physical status score 1 and 2) was conducted between 1976 and 1988.[5] The reported death rate attributable to anesthesia in healthy patients was about one in 200,000 operations.[6] After instituting modern standards of patient monitoring, this same author reported *no deaths* over a three-year period in 244,000 healthy patients undergoing anesthesia and surgery.[7] Other studies confirm that the risk of anesthesia is extremely low in a healthy population undergoing nonemergency surgery if modern standards of anesthesia care are followed by a trained anesthesia specialist.

The Factors Affecting Your Risk of Anesthesia and Surgery

What did anesthesiologists learn from the studies of anesthesia mortality? We learned that assigning an individual patient a numerical risk of anesthesia is difficult, if not impossible, because there are so many factors that influence risk. Your risk of anesthesia depends on a variety of factors related to your underlying diseases, the surgery you are having, and your anesthesia. In fact, your risk of anesthesia will differ from surgery to surgery depending on these factors. For example, if you have high blood pressure, diabetes, and coronary artery disease, your risk will substantially differ if you are having a hernia repair versus if you are having four-vessel coronary artery bypass surgery. Add to the equation other factors that influence risk, like the location where you are having surgery, the credentials of your anesthesia caregiver, and the credentials of your surgeon.

Risk and the Extremes of Age

A few words on the extremes of age and risk are warranted. Many studies suggest that risk increases with advanced age. However, if the elderly patient is in generally good health, or if his coexisting medical conditions are well managed, then the risk of anesthesia and surgery may not be increased. The risk is more related to the patient's biological age and fitness, not strictly chronological age. Conversely, several studies have confirmed that the pediatric patient is at higher risk of complications than the older child or adult and that this applies to the healthy infant, not just the sick.

What You Can Do to Reduce Your Risk

So the question becomes, Can you do anything to influence your risk (or your child's risk) of anesthesia and surgery? You may be surprised to find out that you may be able to reduce your risk—or your child's risk—severalfold. The more coexisting diseases you have and the more invasive and/or specialized the surgery, the more important it is that *you* take charge and influence your risk.

Managing Your Health Before Surgery

Studies of morbidity and mortality associated with surgery and anesthesia during the past fifty years have consistently shown that patients with significant medical problems coming to surgery are more likely to have complications during and after surgery. You need to have your medical conditions optimized before surgery. *Do not accept a battery of tests ordered by a physician or a nurse practitioner in the office as a substitute for good management of your medical conditions.* If you have high blood pressure, diabetes, cardiac disease, or lung disease, have these conditions in their best possible state prior to surgery. This alone can reduce your risk several fold.

Risk of Anesthesia and Surgery and the Importance of Location

The location where you have your surgery does matter. The facility where surgery is performed is extremely important when it comes to high-risk patients and complex or highly specialized surgery. Mortality and complication rates have been shown to vary widely from institution to institution on such major cases as cardiac surgery and major vascular surgery.[8] The evidence suggests that mortality rates for certain complex surgical procedures (e.g., open-heart surgery, major vascular surgery, and total hip replacements) are significantly reduced when the number of cases being performed exceeds a certain minimum number of cases.[9] The same principle holds true for other invasive and complex surgeries. For example, if you are having a liver transplant or a kidney transplant, it may be worth the extra distance to go to the surgeon and a facility that does this procedure on a regular basis in large numbers.

Your managed-care plan may try to send you to a facility that does ten liver transplants a year or thirty-six open-heart surgeries per year because that hospital and/or the surgeon offered the insurer the best financial deal. In my opinion, I would not accept this as satisfactory. The literature suggests that it may be substantially riskier for you to have your heart surgery in an institution that does less than 200 operations per year or your total hip replacement at a facility that does only twenty-five per year. The assumption is that the managed-care company is either unaware of this literature or that it is more concerned about the cost savings than the added risk this may present to you.

The pediatric patient is at special risk during anesthesia and surgery. I would bring my child only to a facility that regularly cares for children and has a staff trained in pediatric care. The problems of children are entirely different than adults, and the way these problems are managed in children are different. This applies equally to inpatient and outpatient pediatric surgery and anesthesia. If your insurance plan sends you to a facility that only occasionally cares for pediatric patients, I would inform the company that the literature suggests this may not be the best care for your child.

Your Surgeon and Risk

The experience of the surgeon doing your operation or your child's operation does make a big difference in your outcome. There are studies that show that complication rates for the occasional pediatric surgeon are higher than the pediatric surgeon specialist, even for operations as simple as a hernia repair.[10] This becomes more significant as the child becomes younger and the surgery more invasive.[11] Based on my observations as a pediatric and cardiac anesthesiologist for more than twenty years and based on the scientific literature, *I would only allow a pediatric surgeon specialist to operate on my child.*

Anesthesia in the Office and Risk

Even if you are healthy, the location where you have your surgery and anesthesia does matter. A serious question has arisen regarding the safety of having anesthesia in the office (*office-based anesthesia*). There have been a rash of deaths in young healthy patients receiving anesthesia in a variety of office settings reported in the literature over the past several years. Office-based surgery and anesthesia often operates below the radar screen of most accrediting agencies and quality review processes that are required of accredited facilities. Before you agree to have surgery or anesthesia in an office-based surgery facility, please read Chapter 28 in its entirety. Please acquaint yourself with the problems that have been associated with office-based anesthesia and surgery and how you can evaluate the safety and quality of the facility before you agree to have surgery there.

Anesthesia Provider and Risk

The credentials of your anesthesia provider may profoundly affect your risk. Studies of mortality associated with anesthesia in the United States and abroad have dropped dramatically over the past fifty years in proportion to the influx of anesthesiologists directing anesthesia care and the elimination of nonspecialists from the anesthesia care team. Nonspecialists administering anesthesia are associated with a higher risk of anesthesia administration than physician anesthesiologists.[12] This subject is discussed in detail in Chapter 1.

Conclusion

The risk of anesthesia in the United States today is far lower than it has ever been. The single most important reason is the dramatic increase in highly trained anesthesia specialists. Other factors decreasing risk are safer and better anesthesia drugs, better and safer equipment to administer anesthesia, and far better patient monitoring. Statistically, in the hands of a trained anesthesia specialist using standard-of-care monitoring and modern equipment and following recommended safety guidelines, the risk of anesthesia to you is exceedingly low. In less than expert hands, or in a facility that is ill equipped to handle your special needs, and under conditions where normal safety standards are not followed or enforced, this could be one of the most dangerous things you or your child will be subjected to.

20

What Are the Potential Complications of General Anesthesia?

Although there are an infinite number and variety of complications that can occur in association with the administration of anesthesia, most are minor and transient. The vast majority of anesthesia complications will require no specific therapy; nor will they interfere with your recovery. It is difficult to estimate the true incidence of complications associated with anesthesia, because most are of such minor nature that they aren't reported. For example, there is no reporting mechanism for a bruised lip or a sore throat from inserting an airway device. These are relatively common complications that lead to no significant harm or debility in the vast majority of patients.

The incidence of more severe complications associated with anesthesia varies from study to study depending on the definition of *severe*. One study reported that severe complications associated with anesthesia were one in 170 anesthetics.[1] But in this study,

headache following spinal anesthetic was listed as a severe complication. In another study, the incidence of *major* complications
associated with anesthesia was reported at one in 731 cases.[2] In
both these studies, the majority of patients who suffered either
severe or major complications from anesthesia still fully recovered
from the injury.

Put simply, any classification system of complications is subjec-
tive and arbitrary. Complications can be classified as major, intermediate, or minor. Consent forms for anesthesia administration
often list the most common and the most severe possible complications associated with anesthesia. Below is a typical listing of the
potential complications from anesthesia that you might see on the
anesthesia consent form before surgery.

Minor Complications Associated with Anesthesia

Minor complications are the most frequent of complications associated with anesthesia. The most common of these are backache
and headache, dental damage, minor eye injury, inability to reverse
the effects of anesthesia drugs, nausea and vomiting, and sore
throat.

Backaches and headache are common in *all* adults, even those
who do not have surgery and anesthesia. Backache is common after
surgery and anesthesia as well. The pain is likely related to lying flat
on your lower back for prolonged periods during surgery, causing
lumbar spine strain. Rarely, a headache may result from a spinal or
an epidural anesthetic (see Chapter 26).

Dental damage is *not* common, yet it is the most common
anesthetic complication resulting in a medical malpractice suit

against the anesthesiologist. Dental damage can be the result of the placement of any type of airway device during general anesthesia. Sometimes, either through operator inexperience, unusual airway anatomy, and/or poor dental condition (loose or damaged teeth, artificial teeth, etc.), a tooth may become dislodged or damaged during an anesthetic.

Eye injuries related to anesthesia are not rare, but they are usually minor. The most common in this category would be a corneal abrasion (scratch). Corneal abrasions occur because the anesthetized patient has no protective eyelid reflex, and thus anything that brushes against the eye may pull back the eyelid and scratch the cornea below. The patient's eyes must be protected while they are anesthetized. The customary technique is to put sterile oil-based lubricating ointment in the eyes and/or tape the eyes shut during the case. Permanent eye injury or blindness can occur during anesthesia due to direct trauma or sustained direct pressure, but this complication is extraordinarily rare.

Inability to reverse the effects of anesthesia usually refers to prolonged effect of muscle-paralyzing drugs. Sometimes, either due to abnormal metabolism in the patient or excessive doses given by the anesthesia caregiver, the effects of muscle-paralyzing drugs cannot be reversed at the end of surgery. If this were to occur to you, the anesthesiologist would place you on a mechanical ventilator until the effects of the paralyzing drug have worn off.

You may have nausea and vomiting following anesthesia, but usually it is mild and short-lived. This is discussed in chapter 22.

You may experience a sore throat after anesthesia regardless of what type of airway device was used during the surgery. If you do experience a sore throat, it is usually mild and resolves within twelve to twenty-four hours without any specific treatment.

Intermediate Complications Under Anesthesia

There are complications occurring during anesthesia that are more serious than those listed above, but in most cases the effect will be transient and you will still most likely have a complete recovery.

Allergic reactions during anesthesia are usually mild and easily managed. These reactions can be seen with the administration of various medications, especially antibiotics, associated with surgery. Allergic reactions in the operating room are increasingly associated with the use of latex products (like gloves). Severe allergic reactions (anaphylactic reactions) are uncommon. Allergic reactions vary in intensity from mild redness of the skin and rash to a full-blown anaphylactic reaction with severe respiratory distress, wheezing, generalized hives, and cardiovascular collapse.

Aspiration pneumonia may occur under general anesthesia when contents from the stomach rise into the back of the throat, and due to the absence of airway reflexes in the anesthetized patient, these contents may be inhaled into the lungs (see Chapter 4). This is *potentially* a very serious complication, but in most cases it is not severe and can be easily treated. In its most severe form, aspiration can lead to overwhelming pneumonia, respiratory failure, and even death.

Awareness is the condition of being awake during surgery when your anesthesiologist thinks you asleep. This is discussed in detail in Chapter 16.

Bronchospasm is a condition where the smooth muscles in the airways constrict and is clinically manifested by wheezing. These constricted airways result in an impaired ability to breathe and exchange gases in the lungs. Bronchospasm can be induced by anesthesia, especially in individuals with a history of asthma or chronic lung disease. This is usually easily treated, but on occasion it can be a life-threatening problem.

High blood pressure and low blood pressure have a variety of causes in the anesthetized patient. Most of the time, these changes in blood pressure are transient and have no adverse consequences. High blood pressure may reflect poorly controlled preexisting hypertension or the stress response during surgery. High blood pressure can stress the heart and increase the risk of stroke. Low blood pressure may be the result of anesthetic induced cardiac depression, hemorrhage, or inadequate fluid replacement. In the patient with poor cardiac function, certain anesthetic agents may cause dangerously low blood pressure. Modest levels of decreased blood pressure are acceptable; profound drops in blood pressure jeopardize most organs of the body, especially the heart and brain.

Nerve injuries associated with anesthesia and surgery may vary from mild tingling in the fingers to complete paralysis. Most nerve injuries are due to patient positioning errors that compress or stretch nerves for prolonged periods of time while the patient is asleep.[3] During normal sleep, humans continually move and adjust body position to keep undue pressure off any particular area. Under general anesthesia, the patient is unaware and unable to move or adjust body position to relieve sustained pressure on a nerve. If a nerve is compressed or stretched long enough, injury will result. Fortunately, most nerve injuries are temporary, and full recovery can be expected in a matter of hours, days, or weeks. Nerve injuries associated with spinal or epidural anesthesia are rare and are discussed in Chapter 26.

Shivering after surgery is common and is often related to the combined effects of anesthesia gases on the central nervous system (especially the spinal cord) and to lower-than-normal body temperature (hypothermia). A variety of factors during surgery and anesthesia may contribute to shivering: To begin with, general anesthesia will significantly inhibit the body's ability to maintain normal temperature; the operating room temperature is frequently frigid; room-temperature solutions are applied to you to cleanse a wide margin around the area of your surgery; and often, large parts of your body are exposed during surgery. When your body temperature drops below normal, your brain responds by having your muscles shiver in an attempt to generate heat. Shivering results in dramatically increased oxygen consumption and activation of the body's stress response. Shivering can actually be dangerous in patients with coronary artery disease and in infants and small children.

Major Complications Associated with Anesthesia

Any of the minor or intermediate complications discussed above might be considered major complications when they occur in their most extreme form. In addition to those, the three most serious complications associated with anesthesia are brain damage, cardiac arrest, and death. Brain damage, cardiac arrest, and death are the final clinical manifestations of a variety of catastrophic events. For example, cardiac arrest may be the clinical manifestation of anesthetic overdose, failure to deliver adequate amounts of oxygen to the patient, or profound blood loss during surgery. These same causes may result in either brain damage or death.

Brain damage by definition includes everything from mild stroke to a full-blown coma. It is rare but clearly catastrophic. The most common cause of brain damage under anesthesia is the failure to adequately ventilate the patient with oxygen. Profound decreases or increases in blood pressure, especially in the fragile, elderly patient, are associated with strokes. Strokes associated with anesthesia are rare except in the extreme elderly who are already at high risk of this complication.

There are three common causes of cardiac arrest related to the administration of anesthesia: failure to adequately ventilate the patient with oxygen, anesthetic overdose, and inadequate fluid replacement. Cardiac arrests are more common in patients with significant coexisting diseases, when the surgery was performed on an emergency basis, and with infants and young children. The risk of cardiac arrest in the pediatric patient is several times higher than the older child and the adult.

Death due to anesthesia is an extraordinarily rare event in a patient having anesthesia with a trained specialist observing all recommended standards of care. Risk of anesthesia is discussed in Chapter 19.

Conclusion

Complications associated with anesthesia are not rare, but most are relatively minor and will lead to no long-term patient harm. With proper monitoring and a properly qualified anesthesia caregiver administering the anesthesia, catastrophic complications associated with anesthesia should be exceedingly rare.

PART III

After Surgery

21

Who Watches Me After General Anesthesia? Does It Really Matter?

Most people assume that once the surgery is over and they are taken to the recovery room that the risk of complications or untoward events is over. Nothing could be further from the truth. In several large studies on complications associated with anesthesia and surgery, a common theme emerges: A significant number of postoperative complications will occur shortly after surgery and anesthesia.[1] In one large study, 42 percent of all complications associated with anesthesia occurred after surgery.[2] Almost half occurred within the first hour following surgery. Most problems were due to inadequate supervision or inadequate management of the patient waking up from anesthesia.[3] The period after anesthesia and surgery clearly should be a period of continued high vigilance. Good postoperative care matters.

Some of the most common problems observed in recovery rooms are airway and respiratory problems. Airway obstruction and inadequate respiration from the effects of residual anesthesia or muscle-paralyzing drugs can be life-threatening if not recognized and promptly treated. You are at risk from other problems as you awaken from anesthesia as well. Commonly seen recovery-room problems are high blood pressure, low blood pressure, bleeding related to the surgery, cardiac problems in the patient with pre-existing cardiac disease, and nausea and vomiting.

These problems are not limited to hospitalized patients receiving general anesthesia; outpatients recovering from anesthesia and surgery have similar rates and types of complications requiring intervention.[4] The patients who have problems and are at risk after a procedure are not limited to those who have received general anesthesia. Patients who have received potent sedative and hypnotic drugs, often called *twilight anesthesia* (see Chapter 25), are also at risk for complications after the procedure.[5] These patients also require proper monitoring and competent observation until they are fully conscious.

The Postanesthesia Care Unit

The recovery room is now usually referred to as the *postanesthesia care unit*. The PACU is where you will be taken immediately after surgery and anesthesia for observation and monitoring by specially trained staff. On arrival, you are given an oxygen mask and connected to many of the same monitors that were used in the operating room. The anesthesiologist will give an abbreviated medical history to your PACU nurse, including your medication history, allergies, type of anesthesia given, surgery performed, and any unusual events that may have occurred in the operating room during the case. Details like blood loss, urine output, and quantity and time of any narcotics administered will also be reported to the PACU nurse.

The PACU nursing staff includes specialists who are trained to recognize and treat the particular and sometimes life-threatening problems you may have while waking from surgery and anesthesia. They are also trained in the effective treatment of pain after surgery. Your anesthesiologist usually fills out an order sheet for postoperative pain medication and for medication for nausea and vomiting, if required. Generally, the anesthesiologist will continue to be responsible for you during the stay in the PACU. The PACU is strategically located near the operating room to ensure the immediate availability of a physician, usually the anesthesiologist, for immediate consultation and response should you have a problem.

When Is It Safe to Leave the PACU?

Criteria for discharge from the recovery room will vary depending on whether you are having outpatient or inpatient surgery. Length of stay depends on how well you are recovering and follows flexible guidelines. Exact criteria will vary, but guidelines that should be met for discharge from the PACU include:

- Absence of adverse events associated with surgery
- Level of consciousness consistent with the return of airway reflexes.
- Ability to maintain an airway without assistance
- Stable vital signs
- Acceptable cardiac, renal, and respiratory function

When you meet these criteria, you can be discharged to the surgical floor, the intensive care unit, or home in the case of outpatient surgery. It is important a competent individual (usually the

PACU nurse) evaluates you prior to discharge to be certain you meet these criteria.

What You Should Know

First, the standards of postanesthesia care for observation and monitoring following general anesthesia or twilight anesthesia should be the same whether the procedure was performed in a hospital, an ambulatory surgery center, or in a doctor's office surgery suite. These standards of postanesthesia care, which apply to all patients who have received general anesthesia, twilight anesthesia, or potent consciousness-altering drugs, have been codified by the American Society of Anesthesiologists.[6] Most accredited facilities follow the ASA standards of postanesthesia care, but many office-based surgery facilities do not.

Second, you or your child should be observed in a setting that has proper equipment for resuscitation, monitoring, assisted ventilation, and oxygen delivery. The PACU should be fully equipped for and able to promptly deal with any emergency that might arise following surgery and anesthesia. A person who is capable of establishing and maintaining an airway and should be available on the premises at all times while you are in the recovery room.

Third, the training and qualifications of the PACU nursing staff watching you or your child recovering after anesthesia and surgery does matter. The person watching you after surgery should be an RN who has been specifically trained as a PACU nurse with appropriate credentials to recognize and treat the problems of the patient in the PACU. This nurse should be dedicated to the PACU area, not performing a supporting role in some other area of the facility (e.g., the operating room). This is a specialized area of nursing similar to critical care nursing where life-threatening problems may occur at any time; many of these problems will require prompt diagnosis and intervention. Your life may depend on the ability of the nursing staff working in the PACU to detect and treat problems that are routine after anesthesia and surgery. In my opinion, all PACU nurses should have advanced cardiac life support (ACLS) training and certification because the treatment of some of the emergencies in the PACU will require these skills.

Lastly, a licensed physician, whether an anesthesiologist or the surgeon (if so qualified), should be on the premises at all times during and after the procedure and available for consultation when you or your child are recovering from anesthesia and surgery until you are ready for discharge.

Conclusion

The recovery period immediately following surgery and anesthesia should be a time of continued high vigilance. There are a significant number of potential complications that can still occur during this period that demands close patient observation and vigilant monitoring by qualified individuals. No matter where you have surgery and anesthesia, you should be properly monitored and observed afterward. Standards of PACU care should apply to all types of anesthesia administered in all venues of practice.

22

Can the Anesthesiologist Prevent Nausea and Vomiting?

Postoperative nausea and vomiting is one of the most memorable experiences patients will ever have of their anesthesia experience. Unfortunately, they aren't good memories. In a study of preoperative anxiety, almost half the patients expressed anxiety about nausea and vomiting after the procedure.[1] Many patients will report they fear nausea and vomiting more than pain. You may feel the same.

Incidence of Postoperative Nausea and Vomiting

The incidence of postoperative nausea and vomiting (PONV) reported in the literature varies tremendously (3–85 percent) depending on the specific patient population being studied, the specific operation being studied, the specific anesthetic technique used, and a host of other factors. The most commonly reported incidence of nausea and vomiting following anesthesia ranges from 10 percent to 30 percent. PONV is the number-one complication in recovery-room patients and is one of the top three reasons for an unplanned admission to the hospital following outpatient surgery.

Factors That Influence Nausea and Vomiting

Body habitus: Obese patients have a higher incidence of postoperative nausea and vomiting than their leaner counterparts. It has been hypothesized that this is due to increased amounts of anesthesia drug deposited in the obese patient's increased fat reservoir. This causes prolonged anesthetic release from fat tissues in such patients after surgery. Obese patients are also at higher risk of nausea and vomiting because they have significantly larger resting stomach volumes and are more prone to the stomach being distended with air during administration of anesthesia.

Gender: Women are four times as likely as men to have PONV. This is particularly true for women in their third or fourth week of their menstrual cycle. There is a significantly higher incidence of nausea and vomiting when gynecological surgery is performed during menses.

Age: The incidence of PONV is greatest in children, especially in the preadolescent eleven- to fourteen-year-old group. At age twenty, the incidence of PONV decreases.

Site of surgery: Surgery performed in the abdomen, especially gynecological procedures, are associated with high rates of PONV. All laparoscopic procedures, which require gas to be inflated in the abdomen (gastrointestinal distension), are associated with higher rates of nausea and vomiting. Eye muscle surgery and ear, nose, and throat surgery (e.g., tonsillectomy) are also associated with a high incidence of PONV.

Location of the surgical procedure: Outpatient surgery is associated with a higher incidence of PONV compared to inpatient surgery because outpatients are required to move sooner (sit up in a chair), ambulate sooner (to leave the facility), and take oral liquids sooner than their inpatient counterparts.

Type of anesthesia agent used: Certain intravenous anesthesia agents are associated with a lower incidence of PONV than inhalation agents (anesthesia gases). This is especially true when the anesthetic agent is Diprivan (propofol). Diprivan is a commonly employed intravenous anesthetic agent with known antinausea properties. Techniques of anesthesia relying on high-dose narcotic techniques will have higher rates of nausea and vomiting postoperatively. The incidence of PONV is substantially lower when spinal or epidural anesthesia is used than when general anesthesia is used. Some studies suggest PONV may occur about one-third as often with spinal anesthesia as with general anesthesia. Nitrous oxide has been implicated in the genesis of PONV.

Duration of anesthesia: The incidence of nausea and vomiting increases with increasing duration of anesthesia and surgery.

History of motion sickness: Patients who give a history of prior nausea and vomiting following anesthesia and surgery or a history of motion sickness are three times as likely to have PONV during subsequent anesthesia and surgery. Early ambulation (motion) following surgery, which is required after outpatient procedures, is associated with a higher incidence of PONV.

Uncontrolled pain: Pain is a common cause of nausea and vomiting and presents a Catch-22. In order to treat severe pain, we often administer potent narcotics. However, narcotics are known to cause nausea and vomiting.

Forcing oral fluids: Forcing the patient to take oral fluids too soon after surgery and anesthesia is associated with a higher incidence of PONV. This is seen most often in outpatients who are offered liquids by mouth shortly after waking.

Preventing PONV

Many of the factors associated with PONV, such as body habitus, age, type of surgery, history of motion sickness, and gender, are usually beyond the control of the anesthesiologist. However, there are many things that the anesthesiologist can do to reduce PONV. The anesthesiologist can prevent the inflation of the stomach with air during the administration of anesthesia or remove it by suction catheter if unable to prevent it. The use of local anesthesia or regional anesthesia at the site of surgery, whenever possible, will lessen the need for narcotic medications after surgery. The anesthesiologist can carefully titrate the anesthesia to the patient using a depth-of-consciousness monitor (e.g., the BIS) to avoid the unnecessary administration of excessive anesthesia. Anesthetic agents known to have antinausea properties may be preferable for outpatients whenever possible (e.g., Diprivan). Diprivan (propofol) is associated with increased direct costs to the facility, but if fewer patients have nausea and vomiting after surgery, those costs will be quickly recovered in shorter recovery-room stays and decreased rates of admission for PONV. Attention to details after surgery are also important, such as minimizing patient movement, avoiding oral liquids too soon, and using nonnarcotic pain medications whenever possible and appropriate.

Treatment of PONV

Even though you might want to prevent or reduce your risk for PONV, prophylactic treatment with the use of potent (and expensive) antinausea drugs on all patients is not justified. About 10–30 percent of all surgical patients will have PONV. If all patients received prophylactic medication for PONV, then seven out of ten patients would receive a drug that was unnecessary. Unfortunately, we cannot determine in advance who will have nausea and vomiting after surgery. If there were absolutely no side effects of these medications, and if they were inexpensive, there might be a case for the routine administration of antinausea medication to all patients prior to surgery and anesthesia. However, these medications are not completely devoid of side effects, and some are quite expensive.

Certain patients *do* deserve prophylactic antinausea medication: those with a strong history of prior PONV associated with anesthesia; patients with history of motion sickness; patients having surgery associated with a very high probability of nausea and vomiting, such as eye muscle surgery, middle ear surgery, gynecological surgery, and laparoscopic surgery; and patients having surgery where vomiting could jeopardize the patient's life (e.g., operations where the jaw will be wired shut and vomiting could result in aspiration of blood and gastric contents into the lungs).

Because there are multiple different causes for PONV, there is no single drug that is 100 percent effective for all patients. There are many drugs touted for nausea, many of which are older and plagued by troublesome side effects, but I will describe only those that are commonly used by anesthesiologists today.

- Serotonin antagonists are a category of drugs that have been around for years, but they were used for their antinausea properties only since the 1990s. The three drugs in this category that are used clinically are Zofran (ondansetron), Anzimet (dolasetron), and, recently, Kytril (granesitron). These drugs were originally used in the treatment of nausea and vomiting secondary to cancer chemotherapy and were an amazing improvement over existing antinausea drugs. These drugs were applied to surgical patients with PONV and were found to be highly effective. Another feature that made them more attractive than previous antinausea drugs was that they are largely devoid of side effects. A small number of patients (3 percent) report headache and dizziness with their use. These drugs represent a remarkable improvement in the treatment of PONV associated with anesthesia and surgery.

- Drugs that cause the stomach to empty are also used in the prevention and treatment of PONV. Reglan is the only drug in this class that is commonly used for PONV. Reglan stimulates gastric emptying and reduces gastric distension—a common mechanism leading to PONV. Reglan occasionally causes the unwanted side effects of uncontrolled muscle spasms and anxiety reactions in some patients. In the obese patient or the patient with decreased gastric emptying from diabetes, Reglan may be useful.

- Scopolamine has been used for many years for motion sickness (e.g., seasickness). Patients with a history of motion sickness can apply a tiny patch that sticks behind the ear that works for up to three days. For the patch to be effective, you must apply it several hours in advance of surgery. Scopolamine is effective for motion sickness, but it also has a high incidence of annoying side effects: dry mouth, sedation, dizziness, spaced-out feelings, light sensitivity, and blurred vision. In elderly patients, it may precipitate psychiatric disturbances and even hallucinations. If you have a history of severe motion sickness, you may ask your anesthesiologist in advance of surgery if this is appropriate for you.

- Droperidol is a drug that was widely used until Zofran and Anzimet replaced it as the drugs of choice for PONV. Droperidol is effective against PONV for up to eighteen hours. The troublesome side effects of this drug (excessive sedation, occasional involuntary and spastic muscle movements, restlessness, paranoia, and dysphoria—a feeling of impending doom) have made Droperidol the poor man's choice for treating PONV.

- Decadron has been shown to enhance the effect of other medications used for PONV and is often given in conjunction with other antinausea medications.[2]

Conclusion

PONV is a relatively common side effect of surgery and anesthesia. With the use of modern anesthesia techniques and short-acting anesthesia drugs with antinausea properties, this complication is often avoided. If not prevented, PONV is usually successfully treated with highly effective antinausea drugs like Zofran, Anzimet, and Kytril. It is important that you notify your anesthesiologist in advance of surgery if you have a strong history of motion sickness or had a prior episode of PONV because you may be a candidate for prophylactic treatment with these drugs.

23

Should I Avoid Narcotic Pain Medication After Surgery?

Many patients will refuse pain medication after surgery or even deny having pain so narcotic pain medications will not be administered to them. A study revealed that more than half the hospitalized patients reported *excruciating pain* after surgery, and almost half these people did not discuss the pain with their nurse or doctor taking care of them. Patient reluctance to take pain medications is common and is most often based on two myths. The first myth is the *fear of addiction* to pain medications; the second is the *no pain, no gain mentality* that pain is somehow good for the body.

Myth No. 1: The Use of Narcotic Pain Medications Will Lead to Addiction

The concern that addiction may occur when treated with narcotics for moderate or severe postoperative pain is quite common, but it is erroneous. Narcotics given in the context of postoperative pain are completely different from narcotics taken to achieve euphoria or taken to satisfy a psychological dependency or addiction.

The scientific literature does not support the myth that narcotics, when given for a short course to treat moderate or severe postoperative pain, lead to addiction.[1] The *recreational* use of narcotics in the absence of pain, or narcotics given over a prolonged period of time, can and do lead to tolerance, physical dependence, and, in rare cases, addiction. Dr. C. Stratton Hill Jr., an expert in pain management, has summed it up: "The patient taking narcotics for pain is trying to get relief from the pain in an attempt to cope with the reality of his or her situation, whereas a drug addict is taking the drug to get out of reality."[2]

The short-term use of narcotics postoperatively in the context of surgical pain only rarely leads to tolerance or physical dependence, and it is extraordinarily rare to lead to addiction.[3] It may take weeks or even months to develop tolerance and physical dependence. It may take years to develop the psychological phenomenon of addiction. The use of narcotics in the postoperative period for moderate to severe pain is totally appropriate and has definite benefits for patients.

Myth No. 2: No Pain, No Gain

The second myth is that pain is somehow intrinsically beneficial. Of course, pain is an excellent defense mechanism when we touch a hot skillet and the pain makes our hand withdraw before we sustain major tissue injury. But pain after surgery is not a bodily defense mechanism serving a beneficial purpose.

Even today there are prevalent negative attitudes associated with the use of pain medications after surgery, as if the need for and use of pain medication somehow represent human weakness.

In contrast to those ideas about the beneficial effects of pain, we now know that persistent pain has many potential harmful effects on the body.

Tissue damage, such as that caused by surgery, causes the release of certain chemical substances locally in the area of injury, as well as direct stimulation of nerve fibers that conduct pain impulses to the spinal cord and then to the higher brain centers that are processed and interpreted as that sensation called *pain*. The body responds to pain in a variety of ways; most adversely affect the body.

Pain leads to a cascade of effects on your body similar to that experienced in the classic fight-or-flight reaction. Stress hormones like epinephrine (adrenaline) are released and can have serious detrimental effects over time if allowed to continue unchecked. The fight-or-flight reaction associated with being frightened lasts a few minutes. The reaction associated with pain after major surgery may last for days. This ongoing stress reaction has a host of negative effects on the body and the psyche when allowed to continue for an extended period of time.

The sustained effects of stress hormones on your cardiovascular system can be serious. Adrenaline release result in an increased heart rate, increased cardiac work, and increased oxygen demand. If you have underlying heart disease, these effects could precipitate angina, heart failure, or a heart attack. The ongoing stress response can also impair your immune response and may substantially increase your likelihood of having complications after surgery.

Severe pain often results in decreased mobility following surgery. Patients who feel pain whenever they move do not want to get out of bed and ambulate. This puts them at increased risk of forming blood clots in the legs. These blood clots can become dislodged and travel to the heart and lungs causing pulmonary embolism, a life-threatening and sometimes fatal condition.

The effects of pain on your lungs and respiratory system can also be serious. Surgery on the upper abdomen results in painful incisions that cause you to have increased muscle tone, decreased deep breathing, decreased function of the diaphragm muscle, decreased ambulation, and decreased ability to cough. All these factors diminish your ability to clear lung secretions that accumulate after surgery. This may significantly lower the oxygen levels in your blood after surgery as well as increase the chance for lung secretions to become infected and develop into pneumonia.

The harmful effects of pain are not just visited upon your body, either. Some of the most negative effects of pain are psychological. Many patients have a high level of anxiety and fear about pain following surgery. Inadequate pain control postoperatively causes not only fear and anxiety but also anger when inadequately treated. It also causes inability for the patient to sleep, which tends to intensify the effects of the pain.

The Benefits of Good Pain Management

With good pain management after surgery, your stress response is lessened. When pain is controlled, you will take deeper breaths, will cough more readily, and will be willing to get out of bed and walk earlier. These behaviors decrease the risk of lung problems, blood-clot formation in the legs following surgery, and the adverse psychological effects of pain.

Conclusion

Untreated pain serves no protective or beneficial function after surgery and may be associated with serious harmful effects on your body. There are clear physical and psychological benefits seen with good pain management after surgery. You should openly discuss your pain with your doctors and nurses so that they can design an effective pain management strategy for you. Effective pain management will often include the administration of potent narcotics medication. The evidence in the literature and vast clinical experience suggest that addiction to narcotics from the treatment of postoperative pain is extraordinarily rare and is not a valid reason to avoid narcotics.

24

How Will My Pain
Be Managed After Surgery?

In a perfect world, the anesthesiologist, the surgeon, or some other health care professional has discussed with you the expected degree of postoperative pain and the options for its treatment before your surgery. Studies have shown that when you have received good pre-operative education and reassurance that your pain will be promptly and compassionately treated after surgery, you are more likely to have higher satisfaction scores, decreased postoperative pain medication requirements, and a shorter length of stay in the hospital.[1]

Who Will Manage Your Pain After Surgery?

Your anesthesiologist generally manages your pain in the immediate postoperative period in the recovery room with the help of a skilled recovery room nursing staff. However, once you leave the recovery room, it varies from institution to institution as to who will manage your pain and how the process is coordinated. There are four different groups of individuals who are commonly involved in the management of your postoperative pain after discharge from the recovery room while you are in the hospital. These individuals often work together in varying degrees depending on the structure of the pain management service at the hospital and the severity of your pain. The groups include: the anesthesiologist, the surgeon, the nursing staff, and, most important of all, the patient.

Regardless of the structure of the pain management service at your hospital, the approach to your pain and the techniques used to treat it will likely be similar.

Assessing Pain

The first step in deciding on a pain management strategy is for your surgeon, anesthesiologist, or nurse to assess the severity of your pain. The approach to treatment will vary depending on your perceived severity of that pain. Pain assessment tools are used to help quantify your pain. These tools are simple to use and can be helpful. For example, with the pain scale assessment tool used at our facility (see Figure 24.1), you will be asked to rate your pain on a scale of 0 to 10, where 0 is no pain and 10 is the worst possible pain. This scale has six faces associated with different levels of pain, which is helpful for children or the patient with a language barrier who may not be able to verbalize their pain in ways we understand. Your child can point to the face that best describes her emotional state to guide appropriate therapy.

Pain Therapy After Surgery

Nonnarcotic Pain Medications

Tissue injury from surgery results in the local release of various chemicals including prostaglandins that cause redness, pain, and

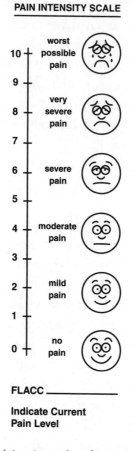

PAIN INTENSITY SCALE

10	worst possible pain
9	
8	very severe pain
7	
6	severe pain
5	
4	moderate pain
3	
2	mild pain
1	
0	no pain

FLACC _____

Indicate Current Pain Level

Figure 24.1   Assessing the Patient's Pain

The patient in pain can point to the face that best characterizes his or her emotional response to the current level of pain.

swelling at the site of injury. Drugs like Motrin, Naprosyn, and Vioxx (*nonsteroidal anti-inflammatory drugs,* or NSAIDS), block a key enzyme in the synthesis of prostaglandins. NSAIDS may be used to combat pain and inflammation associated with surgical tissue trauma. Toradol is a potent and highly effective NSAID commonly used following surgery. Unlike most NSAIDS, Toradol is available in an injectable form, making it rapidly available in the bloodstream. Toradol is comparable in effectiveness to narcotics without the side effects commonly seen with their use. Vioxx is another popular and highly effective NSAID commonly used after surgery.

Local Anesthetics

Local anesthetic drugs (e.g., xylocaine, novocaine, and marcaine) are another class of highly effective nonnarcotic medications that work by a different mechanism of action. Local anesthetic agents are injected into the tissues in close proximity to nerves in the region of the origin of the pain, and they will block the transmission of pain signals from these nerve fibers. This is similar to the injection of novocaine or other local anesthetic agent in your gums at the dentist's office or the injection of local anesthesia before the doctor sutures a laceration. These local anesthetic drugs can block conduction of pain signals from the site of surgery for up to eight to twelve hours after surgery. Local anesthesia at the site of surgery should be used whenever practical to decrease pain postoperatively.

Local anesthetic drugs may also be used to interrupt the pathway of pain at the level of the spinal cord. Impulses from bare sensory nerve endings at the site of tissue injury travel to the spinal cord via small nerve fibers carrying pain signals; they connect with other nerves in the spinal cord (the *dorsal horn*) before the pain signal travels up the spinal cord to the brain. Injecting local anesthesia agents at the level of the spinal cord either by spinal or epidural anesthesia will block incoming pain impulses from being transmitted to the brain. Pain signals will continue arriving from below the level of the epidural or spinal anesthesia, but they cannot be transmitted up to the brain, so there is no perception of pain. For example, continuous epidural anesthesia during labor and delivery using local anesthesia effectively interrupts pain impulses from the uterus during contractions at the level of the spinal cord. The labor contractions continue unabated, but the brain receives no pain signals and the laboring woman perceives no pain.

Narcotics

Narcotics as a family of drugs are also known as *opioids* to indicate their origin from *opium (Papaverum somniferum)*. *Opioids* have been used for pain relief for thousands of years. A host of synthetic narcotics have been created during the past sixty years, with morphine still being the standard against which all others are compared. Potent opioids commonly used in the postoperative patient are morphine, Dilaudid, and, rarely, Demerol. In some cases, a superpotent synthetic narcotic, fentanyl, is used postoperatively. Fentanyl is about 100 times more potent than morphine in relieving pain. These opioids bind to specific sites in the spinal cord and in the brain called *opioid receptors*, where they will attenuate or block transmission of pain impulses.

Weak opioids drugs, like Darvocet and Vicodin, are widely prescribed narcotics for mild to moderate pain following surgery. Codeine is another weak opioid available in liquid form and more commonly used for mild to moderate pain in the pediatric population. You must be able to take medication by mouth, and the gastrointestinal tract must be functioning before this route of administration can be used. Narcotics taken by the oral route result in highly variable blood levels due to unpredictable absorption from the gastrointestinal tract. However, because 65 percent of all surgery is done on an outpatient basis, we must rely heavily on the oral route for the administration of pain medication. Weak opioids will be inadequate for more severe surgical pain.

Strong opioid medications are effective for even the most severe postoperative pain. Potent narcotics can be administered in a variety of ways, limited only by the human imagination. Some methods are more efficient and effective than others in delivering the narcotic to its ultimate destination—the opioid receptors in the spinal cord and the brain. The most common routes of administration of potent narcotics for severe pain are: by injection—either *intravenous* (directly into the bloodstream), *subcutaneous* (into the fat below the skin), or *intramuscular* (directly into the muscle); or by the spinal or epidural route.

Blood levels of narcotic medication following intravenous injection are more predictable than intramuscular injection, which in turn is more predictable than subcutaneous injection. Ultimately, the amount of drug reaching your opioid receptors in the spinal cord and brain depends on the concentration of the narcotic in your bloodstream. If the concentration of the narcotic in your bloodstream decreases, the amount of narcotic reaching your receptors in the dorsal horn of the spinal cord is also decreased, and thus your level of pain relief is decreased. Unfortunately, pain management techniques that rely on the intermittent injection of potent narcotic medications are still commonly employed.

The intermittent injection technique of narcotic administration means that a nurse will administer the narcotic by injection (often intramuscularly) to you every two to four hours. There are several problems with this technique. First, it is highly inefficient for you and the nurse and often results in long delays from the time you request pain medicine and the time it is administered. You must call the nurse and then wait for the nurse to respond. The nurse, often occupied with other patients' needs, must assess your pain, then return to the nursing station or pharmacy to check out the pain medication. The nurse must prepare the injection, return to your room, and inject you with the shot (which hurts). You then must wait up to thirty minutes for the drug to be absorbed from your muscle where it was injected. This is a terribly inefficient, labor-intensive, and time-consuming process that results in narcotic levels in your blood dropping well below therapeutic levels for extended periods of time. This subtherapeutic level of narcotic translates into long periods where you may experience severe pain. There is a much better way.

Patient-Controlled Analgesia

The concept of patient-controlled analgesia (PCA) relies on the belief that *you* are in the best position to manage your own pain.[2] After all, the person experiencing the pain is the only true authority on the existence of the pain and its severity and is the only person in a position to judge the effectiveness of the therapy. The PCA device is a computer-controlled pump that delivers a predetermined dose of narcotic into your intravenous tubing (or even subcutaneously, in some cases) whenever you press a button. This technique of administration rapidly achieves adequate levels of narcotics in the bloodstream. A timer in the PCA box requires that a certain interval of time must pass (the *lockout interval*) before it will allow the delivery of the next dose of narcotic to prevent you from accidentally overdosing yourself.

The PCA is far more efficient, effective, and convenient than intermittent injections for both you and the nursing staff. With

PCA, you have control over the delivery of the pain medication, and there is no delay while you wait for a nurse to respond to your request for pain medication. With PCA, you press a button and receive pain medication directly into your intravenous line on your demand. Following the delivery of the pain medication, you evaluate the effectiveness of the pain medicine and you can administer additional doses of pain medicine if needed. Studies have shown that both patients and nurses give PCA high satisfaction scores. PCA also avoids the painful injections associated with intramuscular and subcutaneous injections. Studies have shown *decreased total narcotic usage* with PCA when compared to intermittent injections.

Not all patients are candidates for PCA. Its use is intended for moderate to severe pain in a hospitalized patient. If a patient is confused, mentally handicapped, too young to comprehend the principles involved, or is likely to abuse the device (e.g., a prior history of drug abuse), then they are not suitable candidates for PCA. The safe use of PCA depends on the fundamental belief that you will use the button only to get relief from pain, not for recreational use or to get high.

Epidural and Intraspinal Opioids for Postoperative Pain

Spinal and epidural techniques may be used for surgical anesthesia as well as long-lasting and effective postoperative pain relief.[3] Generally, only anesthesiologists will use these more complex and invasive methods of pain relief, which are reserved for severe and very severe pain. The administration of potent narcotic medications in close proximity to the place they actually work—the spinal cord's opioid receptors—prevents pain signals at the site of surgery from traveling up to the brain. Because the narcotic (opioid) is being deposited in close proximity to the receptor and is not diluted out in the bloodstream as in other routes of administration, only a tiny fraction of the narcotic dose is required to produce profound analgesia.[4] Unlike local anesthetics, narcotics administered by spinal or epidural routes do not cause muscular weakness or numbness. Use of spinal morphine may produce intense analgesia for eighteen to twenty-four hours. And because an epidural catheter may be left in place virtually as long as we like, epidural morphine can be continued for days if needed.

Side Effects of Opioids

Side effects of opioids are similar regardless of the route of administration: mood changes, sedation, nausea and vomiting, respiratory depression, itching, and, in some cases, constipation. In men, narcotic administration may make it more difficult to urinate. Patients receiving spinal and epidural narcotics need special respiratory monitoring because they may have significant slowing of respirations, sometimes many hours after the narcotic medication was administered. This respiratory depression is easily treated, but it must be recognized. These patients require more vigilance and monitoring postoperatively than is routinely provided, and so these techniques should be reserved for severe pain and employed only when the benefits outweigh the added costs. If the patient is being monitored for respiratory depression, then this technique is safe. If the facility cannot assure this level of nursing care, then the anesthesiologist should not administer narcotics by the epidural or spinal route. It is not appropriate to administer spinal or epidural narcotics to outpatients for acute postoperative pain because such patients are not monitored.

Balanced Analgesia and Multimodal Pain Management

Multimodal pain therapy, or *balanced analgesia*, means that multiple techniques and medications may be used in combination for the most effective treatment of pain.[5] For example, to address the pain associated with a hernia repair, the surgeon might infiltrate local anesthesia at the site of surgery; the patient may receive Toradol (an NSAID) intravenously and be given a narcotic to take by mouth (e.g., Vicodin). The combination of these three modalities is far more effective than any single one. The pathway of pain has many steps, and no single medication or method provides complete pain relief for all patients.

Outpatient Surgery and Pain Management

The desire to decrease the cost of medicine since the 1970s has resulted in the majority of surgical procedures being performed on an outpatient basis. More than 65 percent of all surgeries are performed on an outpatient basis, and those patients are *required* to manage their own pain after they are discharged from the facility. In these cases, the patients must evaluate their pain, decide how much pain medicine is required, and then evaluate the effectiveness of the therapy.

In outpatient surgery, the anesthesiologist and surgeon must proactively deal with postoperative pain. Multimodal pain management is crucial in the outpatient setting. Liberal infiltration of local anesthesia at the site of surgery, early administration of oral narcotic medications, and the administration of Toradol are important for successful treatment of pain in the outpatient.

It is important that you understand the proper dose of pain medicine to take and the *proper dosing schedule* to take it. For moderately painful procedures, the surgeon or anesthesiologist may recommend you take the pain medicine at specified time intervals rather than wait until you are in severe pain. If you wait until you are in severe pain to medicate yourself, often it is difficult to regain good pain relief. Please follow the instructions for the dose and scheduled interval to take the pain medication and ask questions if you are unclear.

Conclusion

First, there are several modalities available for managing pain after surgery that will vary depending on the severity of the pain. Usually, your surgeon and anesthesiologist will anticipate the amount of pain you will have after surgery and discuss pain management options with you. If they don't discuss this with you prior to surgery, please ask them. This will reduce anxiety on your part and will allow you to make an informed decision about your pain management choices.

Second, no single technique of pain management works for all patients. If the technique of pain management being used is not adequately relieving your pain, please notify your nurse, surgeon, or anesthesiologist. Either the dose of medication needs to be adjusted, or additional drugs or techniques may be needed. For the most painful surgeries, we may not be able to get your pain score to 0, but we can usually get it into the tolerable 3–5 range. If your pain scores are consistently 7 or more, your pain management plan needs to be reevaluated.

Third, despite the best plans to proactively manage your pain as an outpatient, sometimes it isn't enough. The most common reason for an unanticipated admission from an outpatient surgery facility is for inability to control pain. If your pain is in the severe and very severe range following surgery despite taking the recommended dose of pain medicine at the prescribed schedule, you may need to be admitted to the hospital for stronger medicine. If the pain seems intolerable, notify the doctor or nurse of this fact. No patient should be sent home or left at home with pain scores in the 6–10 range after surgery. Pain is not good for you, it is not inevitable following surgery, and it should not be continuously unbearable.

PART IV

Types of Anesthesia Other Than General Anesthesia

25

What Is Twilight Anesthesia?

You may have heard the term *twilight anesthesia* in reference to anesthesia other than general anesthesia administered by either an anesthesiologist or a nonanesthesiologist. Although it is widely used, the term *twilight anesthesia* has no standard or commonly accepted definition. The term is ambiguous and confusing, and it may encompass anything from the controlled administration of sedative medication by an anesthesia specialist in the operating room to the administration of potent anesthetic agents by an untrained and unlicensed individual in an office setting to everything in-between. If you have been offered twilight anesthesia for an upcoming surgery, you need to read this chapter carefully.

Twilight Anesthesia and the Anesthesiologist

Twilight anesthesia and general anesthesia have much in common. The ideal skill set of the person who administers twilight anesthesia is similar to the skill set required for those who administer general anesthesia. Anesthesia specialists will sometimes use the term *twilight anesthesia* loosely to refer to a type of anesthesia more correctly called *monitored anesthesia care* (MAC). MAC is the administration of potent sedative and anesthesia drugs by a trained anesthesia specialist, either an M.D. anesthesiologist or a CRNA. It includes the entire continuum of consciousness, from wide awake to a light sleep, using all pharmacological means available to the trained specialist.

The standards of patient care during MAC by a trained anesthesia caregiver are the same as those followed for general anesthesia. During MAC, the anesthesia specialist is in constant attendance during the entire procedure; they use the full complement of patient-monitoring devices that are used during general anesthesia; and they are experts in managing the sedated and the fully anesthetized patient. *It is an axiom among trained anesthesia specialists that sedative medications given during twilight sleep, when given in larger doses or to the patient who is sensitive, will produce a state indistinguishable from general anesthesia.* The anesthesia specialist is always prepared, equipped, and capable of handling the patient who unexpectedly transitions from twilight sleep to general anesthesia.

Twilight Anesthesia and the Nonanesthesiologist

With the dramatic rise in the use of diagnostic and therapeutic procedures requiring sedation outside the operating room, large numbers of patients are receiving potent anesthesia medications by nonanesthesiologists under conditions that are considered appalling and unsafe by most anesthesiologists' standards. There have been numerous documented adverse events associated with the administration of twilight anesthesia by dubiously qualified individuals following unacceptable standards of patient care.[1] Twilight anesthesia can be a freewheeling process in which literally anyone can sedate a patient with minimal supervision, regulation, or peer review because of the mistaken perception that it is so safe.

There may be minor surgeries, but there are no minor anesthetics. When nonanesthesia personnel administer twilight anesthesia, the level of sedation can vary from a patient who is awake, comfortable, and responsive to a patient who is unconscious, unable to maintain an airway, and has lost all airway reflexes. Sedation is a slippery slope without clearly defined borders. Moving from light sedation to deep sedation as described above encompasses a vast continuum of consciousness from a patient who is awake and talking to a patient who is unconscious and unable to breathe without assistance. In practice, this continuum can be crossed in a heartbeat and without warning. In fact, the patient's level of consciousness during twilight anesthesia is often virtually indistinguishable from general anesthesia.

Who's Administering Twilight Anesthesia?

Twilight anesthesia can be administered by a diverse group of individuals, from a fully trained anesthesia specialist to an untrained, unqualified, unlicensed person working in the office or freestanding facility. Outside the hospital setting, twilight anesthesia is essentially unregulated.

In the office-based surgery suite, the nurse circulating in the operating suite most commonly administers the sedation. In many cases, surgeons will administer the sedation themselves.[2] Some surgeons and dentists will use the term *twilight anesthesia* as a euphemism for general anesthesia to avoid medical malpractice liability issues and potential review from state medical or dental review boards. A breast augmentation, liposuction, dental extraction, or laser resurfacing of the face performed under such heavy sedation that the patient only grunts and occasionally writhes on the operating table is not twilight anesthesia; it is an uncontrolled and potentially dangerous general anesthetic.

In dental offices, the dentist or the oral surgeon may administer twilight anesthesia while they are also performing surgery. When the doctor or dentist performing the surgery and the person administering the twilight anesthesia are one and the same person, we have a formula for disaster. In other cases in the office, an unlicensed and sometimes even nonmedically trained individual administers the twilight anesthesia.

Avoiding Adverse Outcomes with Twilight Anesthesia

The adverse outcomes during twilight anesthesia are associated with one or more of the following areas: inadequate preparation of the patient, inadequate training of the provider, and inadequate patient monitoring. In this regard, twilight anesthesia has been a giant step backward in anesthesia safety.

The preparation of the patient is as important during twilight anesthesia as with any other form of anesthesia. The person who administers your twilight anesthesia should be familiar with your medical history and your physical exam, as well as any conditions that may affect anesthesia management and your ability to tolerate the procedure. You should be in your best medical condition possible before the procedure. If you have significant coexisting medical problems, it is even more important that you be in optimal condition, because there is increased risk of adverse events in sicker patients receiving twilight anesthesia.[3] Additionally, because you may slip into unconsciousness with loss of protective airway reflexes at any time during twilight anesthesia, you should fast prior to the procedure to minimize the risk of aspiration pneumonia. Studies report that this safety precaution is widely ignored during twilight anesthesia and is potentially disastrous.[4]

The person who administers your twilight anesthesia should have thorough knowledge of pharmacology of all sedative medications to be used and their possible side effects. Inadequate knowledge of pharmacology is a common factor in adverse events associated with twilight anesthesia. Lack of knowledge of proper dosages of drugs is a common theme and leads to inadvertent patient overdose during twilight anesthesia.[5] In one report, eighty-nine deaths, recorded over a six-year period, were associated with the administration of a commonly used sedative medication by nonanesthesiologists outside the operating-room setting. A majority of the patients died from inadequate breathing after receiving the medication. The individuals administering the drug were not aware that this was a common complication associated with the use of that medication. Not only were these personnel unaware of the potential side effects of the medication; they were also unaware of the simple lifesaving therapy necessary when this occurred.

Airway management skills are an absolute necessity for any person administering twilight anesthesia. Potent sedative medications used during twilight anesthesia will often produce respiratory depression. Inadequate training in airway management has resulted in many preventable deaths during twilight anesthesia. In one case, a child was given potent sedative medications for a minor procedure in the office and stopped breathing. The person who had administered the medications was unable to successfully administer oxygen by bag and mask—a technically simple procedure for an anesthesia specialist—and the child died. In another case, a practitioner administered potent sedative medication to the patient and the patient stopped breathing. There was no oxygen or equipment in the facility available to establish an airway and breathe for the patient, and he died.

Inadequate training in resuscitation skills is another common theme in adverse outcomes seen during twilight anesthesia by non-specialists, especially outside the hospital setting.[6] Numerous adverse outcomes are associated with the inability of the person administering the twilight anesthesia to resuscitate the patient when an untoward event occurs suddenly and without warning. Nonanesthesiologists who administer twilight anesthesia should have the skills to rescue you if you have a problem. These skills are known as advanced cardiac life support.

Standards of monitoring in anesthesia have made an enormous contribution to the increased safety of anesthesia. Monitors are necessary to warn of conditions in the patient that require attention and correction by those who watch over the patient. Lack of adequate monitoring during twilight anesthesia is a common factor linked to adverse events. In one study of adverse events during sedation of children provided by nonanesthesiologists, *the majority of patients were not monitored with a pulse oximeter.*[7] A pulse oximeter is an essential monitor used by anesthesia specialists that continuously measures oxygen levels in the patient and provides early warning of even subtle problems with oxygen delivery and breathing.

The failures in monitoring haven't just been during the procedure, either. There have been several deaths in children associated with the administration of sedative medication at home by a parent who was instructed to do so by the doctor or dentist who would be performing the procedure. The desire was to have a "cooperative" child on arrival to the facility. A number of children have died prior to their arrival at the facility in this way.[8] *It is never acceptable to have a parent administer a potent sedative medication in an unmonitored environment.*

Proper patient monitoring after the procedure is equally important. A competent caregiver at the facility should monitor the patient given potent consciousness-altering drug or twilight anesthesia until the effects of the medication have sufficiently worn off and the patient's level of consciousness is suitable for discharge. A number of patients who have been discharged from a facility following twilight anesthesia before they were adequately recovered from the effects of the sedative medication died either in the car on the way home or shortly after arriving at home.[9] *It is never appropriate for you or your child to be discharged in a semiconscious state from the facility where you received potent sedative medications.*

Standards of monitoring similar to those used by anesthesia specialists during MAC as described above are essential during and after the administration of potent sedative medications, but monitors alone do not protect patients from harm. Monitors only warn of conditions present in the patient. If the person watching the monitor is unable to correctly interpret the information, place it in proper context, and respond appropriately to that information, then you are still at risk. There are documented cases of patients who were monitored appropriately during a procedure but died because the person observing the monitor was unable to properly interpret the monitor, intervene on behalf of the patient, and rescue the patient.[10]

What You Should Know Before You Agree to Twilight Anesthesia

Your twilight anesthesia provider should:

- Be familiar with your medical history and your physical exam, as well as any conditions that may affect anesthesia management and your ability to tolerate the procedure.

- Fully understand the pharmacology of all sedation medications that will be used and their potential adverse effects. This includes detailed knowledge of drug doses, their side effects, and proper treatment for any adverse reaction you may have. In guidelines for administering sedation by nonanesthesiologists, it is recommended that a dedicated trained person *who is not assisting in the procedure* should administer the sedative drugs and monitor you during the procedure.[11]

- Properly monitor your response to the sedative medications during and after the procedure. This person should to be able to correctly interpret and respond to the information provided by the monitors.

- Possess the skills to establish an airway and ventilate you by bag and mask and rapidly establish an artificial airway if necessary. This person would ideally be ACLS-certified.

Also remember:

- It is never acceptable or appropriate for anyone to ask you to administer a potent sedative medication to your child in an unmonitored environment.

- It is never acceptable or appropriate for you or your child to be discharged from a facility where you received potent sedative medications in a semiconscious state.

Conclusion

Twilight anesthesia may transition into general anesthesia at any time. If you are likely to lose consciousness during the procedure, or if you would *like* to be unconscious during the procedure, you should have a trained anesthesia specialist caring for you. For those procedures performed under twilight anesthesia by a nonspecialist, there should be uniform standards of patient care, uniform standards of provider training in airway management and resuscitation, and uniform standards of monitoring—regardless of the venue where the procedure is performed.

26

What Are Spinal and Epidural Anesthesia?

Most people are familiar with the terms *spinal anesthesia* and *epidural anesthesia*. Both methods are safe and offer many advantages over general anesthesia for certain surgical procedures. Yet many patients still have a great deal of fear and misunderstanding about these techniques. You may be one of these people. *Regional anesthesia* is a term used by anesthesiologists to collectively describe epidural and spinal anesthesia and to denote that anesthesia is confined to a region of the body. Regional anesthesia can be used as a complete anesthetic for a wide variety of surgical procedures on the lower abdomen or lower extremities. Regional anesthesia can also be used for surgery in the upper abdomen and even thorax, but in these cases you may require general anesthesia to supplement the regional technique. The use of regional anesthesia is not confined to the operating room either. The use of spinal and epidural narcotics for long-lasting pain relief after surgery is common (see Chapter 24). The use of epidurals for extended pain relief in women in labor is one of the most popular uses for an epidural outside the operating room.

The Difference Between Spinal and Epidural

Despite their many similarities, the spinal and the epidural have significant differences. First, the anatomical location of the epidural space and the spinal fluid are different. The epidural space is approximately one or two millimeters shy of the membrane that contains the spinal fluid bathing the spinal cord (the *dura mater*). The proper placement of the epidural needle is just outside the dura. This is where medication is deposited in epidural anesthesia. For the spinal, we intentionally penetrate the tough dura mater membrane with the spinal needle and enter the space where the spinal fluid is contained. This is where medication is deposited in spinal anesthesia.

The second difference is the equipment used. To place the spinal anesthetic, we use a specialized fine needle with a diameter only slightly larger than a horsehair. This hollow needle is advanced between the bony spines of the vertebral column in the lumbar region of the back and advanced until it penetrates the tough dura mater membrane. When the dura is penetrated, spinal fluid returns through the hub of the hollow needle; then, either local anesthesia or narcotic medication can be injected, and the needle is removed.

For epidural anesthesia, a larger hollow needle, somewhat larger than an adult intravenous needle, is required. The epidural needle is advanced between the bony spines of the lower lumbar region of the back—just like the spinal—except we stop the needle advancement just outside the dura mater, in a location called the *epidural space.* Once the hollow epidural needle is inside the epidural space, a slender, pliable plastic catheter about the diameter of a mechanical pencil lead is fed through the hollow epidural needle and into the epidural space, where it remains after the epidural needle is removed. This resilient, pliable plastic epidural catheter will remain in the epidural space to administer either local anesthesia or narcotic medication for as long as desired.

The third major difference between the spinal and the epidural is the *duration* of its usefulness. The epidural catheter can be used to administer either local anesthesia or narcotic medications literally as long as we choose. In cases of administration of narcotics via the epidural for postoperative pain relief, the catheter may be left in place for several days. In laboring patients, the epidural catheter is routinely used for six to eighteen hours or more for continuous relief from labor pain. There is no fixed time limit on how long the epidural can be used.

The duration of a spinal anesthetic is limited because it is a *single-shot technique.* Once the medication, whether local anesthesia or narcotic medication, is deposited into the spinal fluid, there is a fixed amount of time that it will work. Local anesthetics commonly chosen for spinal anesthesia may last two to four hours or more. A dose of narcotic medication deposited into the spinal fluid may provide excellent pain relief for fourteen to twenty-four hours.

The last important difference between spinal anesthesia and epidural anesthesia is the amount of drug required to establish surgical anesthesia. Epidural anesthesia requires approximately ten times the amount of local anesthesia as spinal anesthesia to establish surgical anesthesia. Likewise, epidural narcotics must be administered in about ten times the dose of spinal narcotics to achieve similar pain relief.

Patient Fears Associated with Spinal/Epidural Anesthesia

If your surgery is appropriate for spinal or epidural anesthesia, and if you are suitable for the technique and no contraindications exist, often you will be offered the option of regional anesthesia. It is common for patients to have a visceral reaction at even the suggestion of spinal or epidural anesthesia. This is not an unusual reaction, but most fears associated with spinal and epidural anesthesia are unfounded.

Fear of being awake during surgery—even if completely pain-free—is a common concern among patients. Except in the case of women in labor or during cesarean section prior to the delivery of the baby, there is no reason that a patient having surgery under regional anesthesia cannot receive adequate sedation during the procedure to eliminate any situational anxiety.

A fear that the insertion of the spinal or epidural needle into the back will be excruciatingly painful is another commonly expressed concern of patients. Except in labor and delivery, where a premedication is rarely given prior to placement of the epidural because of fetal considerations, most patients choose to be heavily sedated prior to the placement of the regional anesthetic; the vast majority will not recall any part of the spinal or epidural placement.

After sedation has been administered to you intravenously, local anesthesia is infiltrated over the spot on your back where the spinal or epidural needle will be inserted (usually the lower lumbar region) so that the area will be numb. The spinal needles used today are about the size of a horsehair. The epidural needle is larger than a spinal needle, but because the local anesthesia has made the area numb, the epidural needle should cause you minimal discomfort.

Another fear is that regional anesthesia will fail and that you will feel the entire surgery. The anesthesiologist should always be prepared to administer a general anesthetic whenever regional anesthesia is used because there is a small chance that the regional anesthesia will be inadequate for surgery. If the regional anesthesia is inadequate for surgery, as determined by a test *before* skin incision is made, then the anesthesiologist may transition to a general anesthetic. Every patient scheduled for surgery under regional anesthesia should be told that general anesthesia may be required if the regional anesthetic is inadequate.

The fear of a *spinal headache* is another concern. Spinal headache is the most common complication of spinal anesthesia that requires treatment. The overall incidence is far less than one in 100 patients if the anesthesiologist uses a tiny, pencil-point spinal needle. The cause of the headache is leakage of the spinal fluid through the puncture site in the dura mater membrane where the spinal needle passed. The continuing spinal fluid leak results in low pressure in the hydraulic cushion supporting the brain. This loss of the fluid shock absorber for the brain results in traction on the nerves of the brain and a severe headache.

Spinal headaches are worse upon standing or sitting and are relieved by lying down. Occasionally, patients have other symptoms as well, including double vision, ringing in the ears, and extreme sensitivity to light. Sometimes the spinal headache does not appear for one to two days after the spinal was performed. Spinal headaches are far more likely in younger patients than older patients. The size of the spinal needle and type of spinal needle used are very important factors in the generation of the spinal headache. Spinal headaches are more common in young female patients, and with the use of larger spinal needles, because the hole in the dura is larger and results in increased spinal fluid leakage.

Spinal headache is quite rare in patients who are more than fifty years old.

A spinal headache may rarely occur following the placement of an epidural as well. If the anesthesiologist inadvertently pushes the larger epidural needle too deep while placing the epidural, it will leave a substantial hole in the dura membrane and a large spinal fluid leak. This is called a *wet tap* in anesthesia lingo. This will almost certainly cause a spinal headache requiring therapy because the epidural needle creates a much larger hole in the dura membrane than the spinal needle.

Symptoms of a spinal headache do not interfere with normal activity in about half of the patients. About one-third of the time the headache is severe enough to limit activity, and the patient will need to lie down periodically to relieve headache symptoms. More than 80 percent of the patients who have a spinal headache will feel better with conservative therapy within five days. Conservative therapy for spinal headache includes pain medicine, rest, hydration, and intravenous or oral caffeine. The remaining patients are incapacitated by the headache and may benefit from treatment.

Treatment of spinal headache is invariably effective. For those patients who have an incapacitating spinal headache or those who do not get better with conservative therapy within forty-eight hours, the anesthesiologist can perform an epidural blood patch (EBP). With the EBP, the anesthesiologist removes a syringeful of the patient's blood from an arm vein under sterile technique and injects this blood into the epidural space above the spinal needle puncture in the dura. This blood forms a patch of sorts over the hole in the dura, which prevents further escape of spinal fluid. EBP is almost immediately successful in relieving the headache in more than 95 percent of cases. Patients may complain of some mild low back pain and pressure where the EBP was placed.

The final, and most intense, fear is the possibility of becoming permanently paralyzed—or some equivalent neurological disaster—from spinal or epidural anesthesia. *The fear of paralysis from spinal or epidural anesthesia far exceeds its occurrence.* In the 1940s and 1950s, there were reports of cases of nerve injury and paralysis associated with spinal anesthesia.[1] Some of the cases were bona fide and serious. However, reports published in the early 1950s of large numbers of patients with neurological problems following spinal anesthesia grossly exaggerated the problem.[2] Much of that data were examined and refuted.[3] Yet the intense fear of spinal anesthesia remained for decades thereafter.

Studies on neurological complications following epidural and spinal anesthesia since the mid 1950s have indicated that serious nerve injury and/or paralysis following spinal anesthesia is an exceedingly rare event. One study reported on 10,098 patients who had spinal anesthesia and reported *no* severe neurological complications related to spinal anesthesia in their series.[4] A second large study on this issue repeated some eleven years later *failed to reveal a single permanent serious nerve injury following spinal anesthesia* in some 11,574 patients.[5] More recently there was a comprehensive review of some 65,304 patients who had received spinal anesthesia with currently accepted drugs and techniques, with only one permanent lesion *possibly* related to spinal anesthesia.[6]

Other causes of neurological injury following spinal or epidural anesthesia include trauma during insertion of the spinal needle, which is most often related to operator inexperience and multiple attempts to place the spinal. Bleeding into the space where the spinal fluid is contained is an extraordinarily rare cause of neurological injury except for those patients taking blood thinners (anticoagulants). Eventually, if the bleeding continues and occupies a large enough volume, it will compress the spinal cord and require surgery to decompress. If you have any tendency toward unusual bleeding or if you are on any blood thinners, your anesthesiologist should know about this; she will likely avoid regional anesthesia to avoid any possibility of this complication.

Other Complications Associated with Regional Anesthesia

Nausea and vomiting are seen in a significant number of patients receiving regional anesthesia. Regional anesthesia may result in a drop in blood pressure, especially in the high spinal or epidural block, as is commonly seen during cesarean section. This sudden decrease in blood pressure may cause nausea and vomiting. Treatment of the low blood pressure with fluid or medication often cures the nausea and vomiting.

Rarely, the spinal or epidural anesthesia medication may travel higher than expected. Instead of establishing anesthesia up to the patient's belly button, the anesthesia level rises to the patient's nipples or higher. This *usually* is not a significant problem, but it may result in a sudden drop in blood pressure and may lead to difficulty with breathing due to respiratory muscle weakness. The attentive and competent anesthesiologist can easily handle this situation.

Unexpected Cardiac Arrest During Spinal Anesthesia

No anesthetic technique comes without risk. Reports have appeared in the literature of cases of sudden cardiac arrest in otherwise healthy patients receiving spinal anesthesia.[7] In most cases, the spinal blocks tended to be high, and the patients had been sedated after the placement of the spinal to the point that they were not responsive to the anesthesiologist. In most of these cases, the first indication that the patient was having a problem was the cardiac arrest. Whether this represents a lapse in vigilance by the anesthesiologist in detecting a patient with inadequate ventilation from sedation or critically low blood pressure, rather than a primary cardiac arrest related to the spinal block, is unknown.

When to Avoid Regional Anesthesia

The reasons to avoid epidural and spinal anesthesia are similar. One absolute reason to avoid regional anesthesia is that you simply don't want these types of anesthesia! Other reasons to avoid regional anesthesia include abnormal blood clotting from any cause (the most common reason being that you are on blood thinners); uncorrected fluid deficit (blood loss or dehydration); infection at the site of needle insertion or infection in the bloodstream (introduces bacteria into the spine causing abscess or meningitis); anatomical factors that make the block dangerous or difficult to perform (e.g., extensive prior back surgery or severe scoliosis); and certain progressive neurological diseases.

Conclusion

The use of spinal and epidural anesthesia is associated with many misconceptions and fears. For certain surgeries, regional anesthesia offers many benefits over general anesthesia. The incidence of permanent nerve injuries or serious complications associated with the use of spinal and epidural anesthesia are quite rare.

27

Is Regional Anesthesia (Spinal or Epidural Anesthesia) Safer Than General Anesthesia?

No anesthetic is without risk, yet many family practitioners, internists, and even surgeons believe that regional anesthesia (*spinal or epidural anesthesia*) is safer than general anesthesia for high-risk patients and should be used whenever possible. Many patients will come to their anesthesiologist after speaking with their regular doctor or surgeon upset and confused about this issue. You may be concerned about this issue, too. Although many nonanesthesiologist physicians have strong beliefs and opinions about the relative safety of regional and general anesthesia, let's examine the facts.

Regional and General Anesthesia and Surgical Stress

Surgery can be a major stress on the body. Activation of the body's stress response results in a cascade of events including the release of certain stress hormones, like adrenaline and cortisol, by the adrenal gland. These hormones can be detrimental to the body in a great number of ways when they persist for extended periods. The release of adrenaline alone increases heart rate, blood pressure, and oxygen demands on the heart, which may be harmful or fatal in the patient with advanced heart disease. It also causes elevated blood glucose levels and can impair the immune response, increasing susceptibility to infection.

General anesthesia inhibits this stress response very little, except in the case of certain high dose narcotic techniques, which are impractical for most surgeries. In contrast, spinal and epidural anesthesia significantly inhibits the body's stress response while the anesthetic is working. This effect of regional anesthesia is most significant for procedures on the lower body. Once the epidural or spinal wears off, however, there are few, if any, differences in the stress response from those seen with general anesthesia.

Of course, postoperative pain also affects the stress response.[1] Effective pain control after surgery will lower the body's stress response. In certain cases, epidurals and spinals can be used to manage postoperative pain. In these cases, some of the beneficial effects of regional anesthesia on decreasing the stress response may be extended into the postoperative period. Some other benefits of regional anesthesia are also measurable.

Blood Loss

Several studies have compared blood loss during surgery conducted under general anesthesia versus regional anesthesia. These studies consistently show significantly less blood loss during certain surgeries when performed under regional anesthesia (spinal or epidural) compared to general anesthesia. For elective hip surgery, blood loss under spinal anesthesia averages 30 percent less than blood loss during general anesthesia. Decreased blood loss with regional anesthesia has also been seen during radical prostate surgery, vascular surgery, and hysterectomy.

Blood Clot Formation

The formation of blood clots can be a good thing or a bad thing. When blood clots prevent further bleeding from a surgical incision, this is a good thing. But when blood clots form in the large veins in your pelvis and legs after surgery (deep vein thrombosis), this is a bad thing. If these large blood clots dislodge from the pelvic and leg veins and travel to the lungs (pulmonary embolism), this is a *very* bad thing. Such clots can obstruct blood flow to the lungs, which can be deadly following major surgery. Prevention of this complication has been an area of focus for all major surgery.

Numerous studies have shown that spinal and epidural anesthesia can significantly decrease the risk of deep vein thrombosis in the legs after total hip and total knee replacement, as well as after radical prostatectomy surgery.[2] Some studies suggest this reduction in blood clot formation associated with use of regional anesthesia may be dramatic (as high as 50 percent in total hip replacement) when compared to patients who had surgery under general anesthesia. The incidence of pulmonary embolism was similarly reduced with the use of regional compared to general anesthesia.

The use of spinal and epidural anesthesia is one way to reduce the risk of deep vein thrombosis following surgery. There are many other ways to decrease the risk associated with blood clot formation in the legs in the perioperative period unrelated to the method of anesthesia selected. Inflatable stockings that are applied to the legs and intermittently inflated and deflated *during* and *after* surgery reduce the formation of blood clots in the legs. Another method to reduce blood clot formation after surgery is the widespread use of blood thinners for a short time postoperatively. Blood thinners decrease the tendency of the bedridden patient to form blood clots in the legs and pelvis. The most important method of decreasing this complication is to get you out of bed and moving as quickly as possible after surgery. Good pain management helps here.

Postoperative Neurological Function

Transient postoperative mental dysfunction in the elderly following surgery and anesthesia is common and occasionally severe (see Chapter 18). The reasons are not entirely understood. Although intuitively it would seem likely that spinal or epidural anesthesia would lead to less postoperative mental dysfunction, this has not been demonstrated in most studies on this subject.[3] These studies suggest that the choice of anesthetic seems to have little impact on the mental changes seen in the elderly associated with hospitalization and surgery.

Pulmonary Complications

There are many theoretical reasons why regional anesthesia might be superior to general anesthesia in preserving lung function after surgery. Contrary to conventional wisdom, most scientific studies cannot demonstrate any significant difference in lung function following surgery in patients who had a regional versus general anesthesia. Trends suggest some benefits of regional over general anesthesia in reducing pulmonary complications, mostly by decreasing pain and improving ambulation sooner, but the evidence is *underwhelming*.

Despite a lack of data demonstrating clear benefits of regional over general anesthesia in patients with preexisting lung disease, many anesthesiologists will choose regional anesthesia for their patients with advanced lung disease for surgery on the lower body to avoid the need to instrument the airway. Airway devices, like the endotracheal tube, may significantly irritate the airways in the patient with severe lung disease and stir up a host of unwanted side effects like bronchospasm (wheezing), increased coughing, and straining. Regional anesthesia usually avoids these problems.

Cardiac Complications

It is a reasonable hypothesis that the blunted stress response provided by regional anesthesia during surgery might lead to a decrease in cardiac complications in the high-risk cardiac patient. Unfortunately, numerous studies have failed to demonstrate any significant differences in cardiac complications between regional and general anesthesia in this regard.[4] In fact, most studies have failed to demonstrate any statistically significant differences in mortality rates between patients who received regional anesthesia and those who received general anesthesia.

Length of Stay in the Hospital

There is no significant difference in the length of stay in the hospital for patients who had regional anesthesia versus those who had general anesthesia in most studies that have looked at the issue.

Conclusion

The decision of your anesthesiologist to recommend regional anesthesia is based on many considerations including your preference, the location of your surgery, your risk of deep vein thrombosis, your risk of major blood loss, and the anticipated severity of your postoperative pain. However, a well-managed anesthetic is far more important than the specific technique chosen. If your case is managed well during and after surgery (e.g., prophylaxis against blood clot formation and good postoperative pain management leading to early ambulation and decreased pulmonary problems), this is far more important on your outcome than the specific anesthetic technique chosen in the operating room.

Is It Safe to Have a Procedure in the Doctor's Office Under Anesthesia?

The well-known phrase *caveat emptor*—"buyer beware"—is an appropriate warning for the person contemplating surgery and anesthesia in the office. A patient cannot be too careful when choosing who will do the surgery, who will administer the anesthesia, and where this will occur. Many patients assume that office-based surgery and anesthesia are equivalent in quality and safety to the hospital or accredited ambulatory surgery center facility. This is a reasonable assumption, but it is often incorrect.

Office-Based Surgery

Office-based surgery is defined as any procedure done in a doctor's office, be it cosmetic surgery, aesthetic surgery, plastic surgery, oral surgery, dental procedures, or any other painful procedure that requires the administration of potent consciousness-altering drugs or general anesthesia to accomplish. This does not refer to an injection of local anesthesia to fill a cavity in a tooth, remove a wart, or suture a laceration.

The subject of anesthesia and surgery in the doctor's office has received attention in both the printed and electronic media due to high-profile disasters associated with its use. Many of these disasters have occurred during relatively uncomplicated procedures on young, healthy patients, some involving children. Many of these deaths and complications in the office were related to grossly substandard medical practice. Most of the deaths and complications that have come to public awareness were judged to be preventable if the same standards of care had been followed in the office suite as required in accredited hospitals and ambulatory surgery center facilities.

This is not a trivial issue. Office-based surgery is a significant portion of all surgeries, and its number is growing rapidly. Only crude estimates of the actual number of office-based surgeries exists. In 1984, less than a half-million procedures were done in the office. In 1990, the number was estimated at 1.2 million.[1] In 1996, it was estimated at more than 3.4 million surgeries. You may be considering having surgery in the office as well. If so, please read carefully.

Practitioners who have converted a portion of their office into an operating room say this is done for convenience for themselves and their patients. They cite the decreased facility cost of performing the surgery in their office as a benefit to their patients. For the surgeon, it certainly is more convenient to do the surgery in the office. She can schedule cases any time she wants. At the local hospital or ambulatory surgery center facility, she must compete with other surgeons on staff for time in the operating room.

But this is really about making money. Lots of it. Office-based surgery procedures are extremely lucrative, and currently they are largely unregulated. This is a formula for professional turpitude inspired by greed. Some practitioners see this poorly policed and largely unregulated practice as a cash cow. In many cases, the lack of oversight and peer review in the office has allowed marginal and often unqualified practitioners to perform lucrative procedures they would never be allowed to perform in any accredited facility for lack of adequate training. So, although the direct financial cost for the office-based surgery suite is lower than in the accredited facility, the personal cost to the patient may be substantially more.

As a fundamental rule, medical practitioners and the facilities where they work should conform to uniformly high standards of care. The standards of care should be equivalent whether surgery is done in the hospital, in the ambulatory surgicenter, or in the office surgery suite. Unfortunately, at present there are no enforceable regulations or mandatory standards for office-based surgery suites in forty-seven out of fifty states in this country. Policies and standards of care that are an absolute requirement in the hospital or accredited surgicenter facility often do not exist in the office-based surgery practice. You should evaluate four areas in the office-based surgery suite before agreeing to have a procedure performed there:

1. *The practitioner*: Who will perform the procedure?
2. *The anesthesia*: Who will be giving the anesthesia?
3. *The facility*: Where will the procedure be done?
4. *The ancillary staff*: Who will assist in the care of the patient throughout this process?

The Practitioner: Who Will Perform the Procedure?

When a physician applies for privileges to perform surgery in the hospital setting, a committee of peers will investigate their credentials and training and decide if the practitioner has had the proper training and experience to be granted the specific surgical privileges requested. If the applicant has the proper credentials and performs satisfactorily on supervised cases, he is granted privileges in the specific area of surgery requested. But keep in mind that being awarded privileges in the department of orthopedic surgery does *not* confer privileges in the department of plastic surgery. A physician must show evidence of proper training and competence in each area of requested surgical privileges in order to be granted those privileges.

In office-based surgery, physicians are granted surgical privileges based on the Golden Rule: *The person with the gold makes the rules.* A practitioner may be an obstetrician or orthopedic surgeon by residency training and even have privileges in the department of obstetrics or orthopedic surgery at the local hospital, but in the office-based surgery suite, anyone can declare him- or herself an "aesthetic surgeon" or a "cosmetic surgeon" after a weekend course. In a hospital setting, an orthopedic surgeon or obstetrician who had taken a three-day course in cosmetic surgery would not be considered sufficiently trained to be granted privileges to perform face lifts, breast augmentations, tummy tucks, or liposuction procedures.

It has been estimated that *posers*—persons who pretend to be something they are not—perform about half of all liposuction procedures done in the office. Posers commonly attend two- to five-day courses on cosmetic or aesthetic surgery, which they believe can adequately train them to be competent in various cosmetic surgery procedures. Breast augmentation surgery, laser resurfacing of the face, and liposuction are the three most common procedures that physician-posers think they can master in a few days. Posers were residency-trained to be general practitioners, internists, obstetricians, gynecologists, emergency room physicians, dermatologists, surgeons, dentists, and even anesthesiologists.

The terms *aesthetic surgeon* or *cosmetic surgeon* may be a warning sign for a dubiously qualified practitioner (i.e., a poser). This person may not be trained as a surgeon at all. Some of these practitioners have declared themselves to be "board-certified" cosmetic surgeons after taking a five-day course. They may even have an impressive diploma on the wall of their consultation suite attesting to this fact. To accurately assess the qualifications of your prospective office-based surgeon, ask them if they completed an accredited residency program and what specialty it was in. This will tell you what they were really trained to do.

How many people are damaged or killed by substandard and dangerous practices in the office? We'll never know because the law does not generally require reporting of complications and deaths in the office surgery suite. Medical malpractice claims are only the proverbial tip of the iceberg because many adverse events do not result in litigation. Only a tiny fraction of adverse outcomes appear in the media. Closed medical malpractice claims in Florida have identified 830 deaths and some 4,000 injuries associated with office-based medical practice from 1990 to 1999.[2]

Anesthesia in the Office

Anyone can provide anesthesia in the office. Sometimes it's the surgeon or dentist performing the procedure. Sometimes it's a nurse. Sometimes it's a medical or dental assistant. In a pinch, it has even been the person answering the telephone at the receptionist desk. Sometimes it's a CRNA. Occasionally, it's an M.D. anesthesiologist.

In a survey of aesthetic surgeons performing surgery in the office, the majority said their circulating nurse administered the intravenous sedative medication to the patient, and more than one-third said they administered the medication themselves.[3] Many dentists and surgeons are directing the anesthesia administration by an office employee while they are also performing the procedure. In anesthesia circles, this is known as *anesthesia by proxy*. Sometimes the proxy is an RN, and sometimes the proxy is a dental hygienist with no medical training whatsoever. These anesthesia proxies administer potent anesthesia drugs of which they have little knowledge, and they are often incompetent in managing the life-threatening complications that arise from their use. Many anesthesia proxies are not trained in ACLS and are not certifiably competent in rescuing the patient from an untoward event.[4]

Patients having surgery in the office are often told they will receive twilight anesthesia, often a euphemism for an uncontrolled, poorly conducted, and potentially dangerous general anesthetic. Many of the patients who are told they are going to receive twilight anesthesia are actually completely unconscious and have all the attendant risks associated with general anesthesia without an anesthesia specialist managing and monitoring them.

Anesthesia equipment in the office is often cause for serious concern. Anesthesia machines in the office, if available at all, are often ridiculously outdated. These older machines lack essential safety features of modern machines. Modern anesthesia machines, unlike those that are thirty years old, have a variety of redundant safety features to protect patients from catastrophic harm from simple human error or other hazards. Modern anesthesia machines have safety features that rapidly detect oxygen supply failure (which, by the way, is much more likely to occur in the office than the hospital); a disconnection between patient and anesthesia machine; and inadequate ventilation of the patient. These simple errors, if not detected and corrected rapidly, can lead to brain damage, cardiac arrest, or death in a matter of minutes. These older machines often pollute the operating room and all who work there with waste anesthesia gases because there is no so-called scavenger system to capture and remove gases from the operating room. Using a thirty-year-old anesthesia machine is similar to driving a car with no seat belts, no air bags, and no engine warning lights that is spewing black smoke and pollution out the tailpipe.

Patient monitoring standards in the office appear to be more cavalier than those required in the hospital setting. In a survey given to aesthetic surgeons, 5 percent reported they did not monitor blood pressure, 7 percent did not use pulse oximetry (an essential safety monitor during any anesthetic), and 11 percent did not monitor the electrocardiogram during the procedure.[5] The actual number of patients who are not properly monitored during office-based anesthesia may be higher than quoted in the survey because physicians and dentists with substandard practices aren't the ones who would volunteer this information. Along with the increased number of highly trained anesthesia specialists, improved patient monitoring during anesthesia and surgery is one of the most important reasons anesthesia morbidity and mortality have declined so dramatically since the 1950s.

The Facility Standards

Some office-based surgery suites are disparagingly referred to as *converted garages* to reflect the size and sophistication of the room where the procedures are performed. Many of these "suites" are actually examining rooms that are converted into an operating room when a patient is having surgery. These suites often are missing essential safety features that are required of hospital and ambulatory surgery center facility operating rooms. Treatment rooms in doctors' offices were not intended to be formal operating rooms when they were built. They were not equipped with proper electrical outlets and emergency backup generators as hospitals and accredited ASC facilities are. If power is ever cut off in the middle of office-based surgery, there is often no backup generator.

Proper equipment and supplies are essential in the modern operating room—adequate lighting, properly functioning sterilizers, proper surgical and anesthesia equipment for the procedure, proper attire for the operating room, and so on. There must also be adequate backup supplies of oxygen available for administration to any patient who requires it for as long as they require it. Inadequate oxygen supplies have been a factor in deaths and adverse outcomes in the office-based surgery suite. There have been case reports from office surgery suites where oxygen was either not available during a crisis, or there was inadequate backup supply of oxygen when needed.[6]

Improper sterile technique and improper sterilizing procedures are a common cause of patient harm in the office-based surgery suite. One surgeon in California had more than three dozen patients who acquired serious infections from liposuction procedures because the facility had the habit of reusing disposable equipment and other abhorrent transgressions in surgical instrument sterilization procedures.

Inadequate pharmacy has been a factor in deaths and adverse outcomes in the office-based surgery suite. Dantrolene is an essential drug in the treatment of a rare but potentially fatal reaction that may occur under anesthesia known as *malignant hyperthermia syndrome* (MHS) (see Chapter 9). In any facility where general anesthesia is administered, Dantrolene must be immediately available for treatment of this syndrome should it occur. Unfortunately, many office-based surgery and dental suites where general anesthesia is administered do not stock Dantrolene because it is expensive, it is difficult to store, and only rarely will it be needed. An inadequate pharmacy to treat cardiac rhythm problems has also been reported in the office.

The Ancillary Staff in the Office

The quality of the care you receive is related to the quality of the individuals who provide it. This does not only refer to the surgeon and the anesthesia provider. Often the people working in the office-based facility who will be taking care of you and assisting in the surgery are not trained in the capacity they are working. Sometimes the skill set of the employee does not match the job he is being asked to perform in the office-based surgery suite. The questions you need to ask are: Is the surgical assistant certified by his or her own organization? Are these individuals knowledgeable and formally trained in proper sterile technique? Sometimes untrained individuals are asked to perform these functions but are ill equipped to do so, which may result in an inordinate number of horrific infections. Are the nurses working in the facility trained in ACLS, and are they certified as competent in rescuing you from an untoward event? Will the RN in the operating room be your advocate or the surgeon's lackey? Does the RN understand proper standards of patient care during and after surgery, and is he willing to question the surgeon if those standards of practice jeopardize you?

Some office-based surgery suites *do* adhere to the same standards of care followed by accredited hospitals and ASC facilities, but how can you evaluate which environment is safe and which environment should be avoided? *You must ask questions.* What follows is a list of questions patients should ask and have answered before they will agree to have surgery in the office.

The Questions You Should Have Answered Before Agreeing to Surgery in the Office

The Anesthesia Patient Safety Foundation published a list entitled "Questions to Ask Before Accepting Office-Based Anesthesia."[7] Their comment was that patients should be educated to ask the proper questions to ensure the safety of their individual experience and to provide an incentive to establish a single safety standard regardless of the site where surgery and anesthesia are performed. These are the twenty-two questions from the Anesthesia Patient Safety Foundation:[8]

1. Is your office accredited for performance of surgery and administration of anesthesia?
2. How many of these operations have you performed and would you have this operation in an office such as yours if you were the patient?
3. Are you credentialed to perform this operation in a hospital or accredited ambulatory surgery facility?
4. Who will administer my anesthesia and what are his/her qualifications?
5. Is the individual administering my anesthesia credentialed to administer anesthesia in an accredited hospital or ambulatory surgery facility?
6. Is the individual administering my anesthesia certified by his/her certifying organization?
7. When will I meet the individual responsible for administering my anesthesia?
8. What are the choices available to me for anesthesia?
9. Will the individual administering my anesthesia be in constant attendance with me during my anesthetic?

10. Will the anesthesia machine used for my anesthetic be modern and equivalent to the machine that would be used if I had this operation in a hospital or ambulatory surgery facility?

11. Will the monitors used on me during my anesthetic be the same that would be used if I had this operation in a hospital or ambulatory surgery facility?

12. Do you have the necessary equipment and drugs to handle any possible emergency that might occur during or following my anesthetic?

13. What hospital will I be admitted to should a complication occur during my anesthetic?

14. Is there a separate area where I will be taken to awaken from my anesthetic?

15. What are the qualifications of the individual who will monitor me in this in this recovery area?

16. Will the monitors used during my recovery from anesthesia be the same that will be used if I was recovering after surgery in a hospital or ambulatory surgery facility?

17. Is the recovery area in your office equipped in a similar manner to the recovery area in a hospital or ambulatory surgery facility?

18. Who is responsible for determining if I am ready to be discharged home?

19. Who is ACLS certified in your office?

20. How is the operating room cleaned between cases?

21. How are the instruments sterilized?

22. Is appropriate surgical attire worn by those in attendance during my surgery?

29

The Bottom Line

I hope this book has answered all of your questions about anesthesia and helped you to become better equipped to evaluate your anesthesia caregiver and the facility where it will be administered, as well as to ask the right questions to obtain the best and safest care for you and your child. Everything covered in this chapter has been covered in more detail elsewhere in the book, but I would like to review a few of the most important safety issues, which I call *the Bottom Line*, as a checklist to go through when you or your child are scheduled for anesthesia. These points can be categorized into four areas:

- You and your coexisting diseases
- Your anesthesia caregiver
- The facility where you will have the procedure done
- The person who will be performing the procedure

You and Your Coexisting Medical Diseases

One of the most important things you can do as a patient is to be in your best medical condition at the time of surgery and anesthesia. This can substantially reduce your risk of anesthesia and surgery. This may require very little preparation if you are an otherwise healthy person. However, the more coexisting diseases you have, the more important this is. Do not accept a battery of medical tests ordered by your regular doctor or her office personnel as a substitute for a proper history and physical exam and proper treatment of your medical conditions. If you have high blood pressure, diabetes, heart disease, lung disease, or other medical problems, these conditions should be well controlled and in their best possible condition prior to surgery. *Lab tests do not optimize these conditions, but proper medical care can.* Being in your best medical condition includes being in your best psychological condition as well.

Preparing for anesthesia and surgery also means preparing mentally. If you are psychologically unprepared for surgery or have a psychiatric illness, this should be addressed and treated prior to elective surgery. Elderly patients with excessive anxiety or depression prior to surgery have a much higher rate of postoperative confusion than their elderly counterparts without these conditions. Even healthy patients may experience a serious adjustment disorder or depression after anesthesia and surgery if not properly prepared mentally for the experience. Studies have shown that patients who are better prepared psychologically for surgery have smoother recovery after surgery and require less pain medication. Part of your mental preparation for surgery is a good preoperative meeting with the anesthesiologist.

The importance of a good meeting with your anesthesiologist has been stressed in several places in the book. This meeting is especially important if you have significant medical problems or unusual personal or family history of problems with anesthesia. It is important your anesthesia caregiver is aware of all your medical problems and can anticipate potential problems and be prepared for them. In fact, you should request to speak to your anesthesiologist in advance of surgery if you have *any* questions or anxieties about your anesthesia. This meeting is a chance for you to discuss any questions, fears, and concerns you may have regarding anesthesia. A good meeting with your anesthesiologist has been shown to decrease your anxiety level, your postoperative pain medicine requirement, and possibly even your length of stay in the hospital.

The Anesthesia Caregiver

A recurrent theme in this book is that the quality of your anesthesia provider does matter. The anesthesia caregiver will be monitoring and managing your vital functions during surgery in addition to making sure you are adequately anesthetized for the contemplated procedure. It is essential that the person caring for you is competent to do that. To find out the credentials of your anesthesia caregiver, all you need to do is ask. Anesthesia specialists are proud to tell you the amount of training that was required to become an M.D. anesthesiologist or a CRNA.

Although trained anesthesia specialists are generally competent to administer virtually every type of anesthesia, there are two areas that deserve special mention as areas of substantially higher risk where specialty training and experience may influence how well you or your child does. If you are having open-heart surgery (cardiac anesthesia), or if your child is having surgery (pediatric anesthesia), it would be preferable to have an anesthesiologist who has had specialty training in this area and is performing this kind of anesthesia on a regular basis. Anesthesiologists who are only doing an occasional heart case or occasional pediatric case may not maintain the highest levels of proficiency in these areas. If I am having heart surgery, I prefer an anesthesiologist who is regularly doing cardiac anesthesia at a hospital performing at least 200 heart operations per year (see below). For my infant or child, I prefer an anesthesiologist who regularly anesthetizes infants and children and a facility that regularly cares for infants and children.

If you or your child will receive anesthesia by anyone other than a trained anesthesia specialist, please reread Chapters 1, 25, and 28. You have every right to ask the qualifications and training they have received to perform this function and what type of anesthesia you will receive. Be aware that the term *twilight anesthesia* may be a euphemism for an uncontrolled general anesthetic administered by a marginally trained or untrained individual. If you are sedated for any procedure to the point where you are unresponsive to verbal stimuli or unconscious, you are in a state indistinguishable from general anesthesia. You have all the attendant risks of general anesthesia without the benefit of a trained anesthesia specialist. I personally would not receive general anesthesia from anyone other than a trained anesthesia specialist.

If you are going to receive sedation for a painful procedure or surgery by anyone other than a trained anesthesia specialist, it is essential that you ask questions!

- What are the credentials and training of this person to administer powerful sedative medications?

- Is this person able to recognize the side effects and complications of these medications and prepared to deal with any complications you might have as a result of the administration of these medications? Is this person able to establish and maintain an airway if the need arises?

- Will you (or your child) be monitored during the procedure in accordance with ASA recommendations for monitoring during sedation by nonanesthesiologists?

- Is the person administering the sedative medications dedicated to monitoring you, or will they be participating in other activities that draw their attention away from you? The person administering the sedative medication should be dedicated to monitoring you for the effects and side effects of those medications.

- Is this person certified in ACLS?

Regardless of the procedure or the specific type of anesthesia, it is appropriate for you, the patient, to candidly ask your anesthesia provider if they will be present and paying attention to you during the entire procedure. It is reasonable and appropriate for you to ask your anesthesia provider to minimize all distractions that may divert their attention from you (or your child) during anesthesia.

The Facility

There are important issues regarding the facility where you will have your procedure and be cared for that warrant mentioning one last time. Please ask if the facility where you or your child will have anesthesia and surgery is accredited by the Joint Commission and Accreditation of Hospitals Organization and is accredited for the administration of anesthesia and surgery. Most hospitals and ambulatory surgicenter facilities are required to have this accreditation. If you are having anesthesia in a doctor's, surgeon's, or dentist's office or in a radiology suite, you must be even more vigilant because there is little oversight of those types of facilities by traditional regulatory organizations and few laws governing standards of anesthesia care in these remote locations. You can find a list of questions at the end of Chapter 28 that you should ask and have answered regarding office-based surgery, dental, and radiology suites to evaluate the quality and safety of the facility.

If you are having complex and high-risk surgery, like cardiac surgery, major vascular surgery, or transplant surgery, I recommend that you do some homework before deciding on the facility where to have the surgery. You should ask the number of that procedure the hospital does per year and if there is any published data that compare the results of that hospital to others performing similar procedures. Often these results exist and are available to the public, but patients aren't aware of them. If I required heart surgery, I would choose a hospital that does more than 200 heart operations per year. If I needed a liver transplant or kidney transplant, I would choose the facility that does at least 100 of those procedures per year. Even for total hip replacement surgery and prostate surgery, I would choose a facility that does those procedures in higher numbers (100 per year or more), rather than the facility doing less than that.

The location where your child will have surgery and anesthesia is another area of special consideration. Evidence suggests that the best of all situations is to have your child cared for by a team of physicians and nurses that regularly cares for infants and children. This becomes increasingly important as the child becomes younger and sicker. It may be worth the extra travel and inconvenience to have your child cared for at a facility that regularly cares for children.

The final area of concern worth investigating before scheduling surgery and anesthesia relates to the nursing staff. Many hospitals have downsized nursing staffs to dangerously low levels, resulting in inadequate numbers of nurses caring for patients. This has been shown to result in worse patient care and increased complication rates. The recommended nurse-to-patient ratios should be on the order of 1:5 on a normal acuity floor and 1:2 in the intensive care unit. Fewer nurses per patient means less attention and care from your nurse while recovering from surgery. The sicker you are and the more extensive your surgery, the more important it is that you have a competent nurse who will be available to respond to your needs and recognize problems you may have after anesthesia and surgery.

The Person Performing the Procedure

It is essential you know the credentials of your surgeon. Do not assume he is qualified to perform the surgery you have been scheduled for. This was discussed in detail in Chapter 28 but deserves mention again. Don't accept the diploma on the wall as evidence of competence. Ask your surgeon what his residency training was in. This was what they were formally trained to do. Surgeons are proud of the amount of work they had to do to become surgeons and are not offended by a question about their training. Ask your surgeon how much training was required to obtain that diploma on the wall of their consultation suite. For many aesthetic or cosmetic surgeons operating in their office, it was obtained after a three- to five-day course in cosmetic surgery. This is most problematic in the office-based surgery suites, where there is very little oversight or regulation.

Parting Words

Anesthesia today is safer than it has ever been because of the improved quality of the anesthesia provider, improved patient monitoring, improved safety of anesthesia drugs, and improved postoperative nursing care. If you follow the advice in this book, you have the knowledge to make the safest choices and the knowledge to decrease your risks during anesthesia to the lowest possible number. But remember, this applies only when you have selected a trained anesthesia specialist, using all recommended patient safety monitors, in an accredited facility following all accepted standards of patient care. Knowledge is power! Please use what you have learned in this book to make your anesthesia and surgery experience as safe and stress-free as possible. Good luck.

Notes

Chapter 1

1. Courtiss, E. H., et al. (1994), "Anesthetic Practices in Ambulatory Aesthetic Surgery," *Plastic and Reconstructive Surgery* 93: 792–801.

2. Bechtoldt, A. A. Jr. (1981), "Committee on Anesthesia Study Anesthetic-Related Deaths, 1969–1976," *North Carolina Medical Journal* 42: 253–259; Forrest, W. H. (1980), "Outcome: The Effect of the Provider," in R. A. Hirsh et al., eds., *Health Care Delivery in Anesthesia* (Philadelphia: George F. Stickley), pp. 137–142.

3. Silber, J. H., et al. (2000), "Anesthesiologist Direction and Patient Outcomes," *Anesthesiology* 93: 152–163.

4. Beecher, H. K., and D. P. Todd (1954), "A Study of Deaths Associated with Anesthesia and Surgery," *Annals of Surgery* 14: 2–34.

5. Warden, J. C., and B. F. Horan (1996), "Deaths Attributed to Anaesthesia in New South Wales, 1984–1990," *Anaesthesia and Intensive Care* 24: 66–73.

6. Eichhorn, J. H. (1989), "Prevention of Intraoperative Anesthesia Accidents and Related Severe Injury Through Safety Monitoring," *Anesthesiology* 70: 572–577.

7. Abenstein, J. P., and M. A. Warner (1996), "Anesthesia Providers, Patient Outcomes, and Costs," *Anesthesia and Analgesia* 82: 1273–1283.

Chapter 2

1. Warden, J. C., and B. F. Horan (1996), "Deaths Attributed to Anaesthesia in New South Wales, 1984–1990," *Anaesthesia and Intensive Care* 24: 66–73.

2. Egbert, L. D., et al. (1964), "Reduction of Postoperative Pain By Encouragement and Instruction of Patients," *New England Journal of Medicine* 270: 825–827; Egbert, L., et al. (1963), "The Value of the Preoperative Visit by an Anesthetist," *Journal of the American Medical Association* 185: 553–555.

3. Gaba, D. M. (1989), "Human Error in Anesthetic Mishaps," *International Anesthesiology Clinics* 17: 137–147.

4. Pederson, T., et al. (1990), "A Prospective Study of Mortality Associated with Anaesthesia and Surgery: Risk Indicators of Mortality in Hospital," *Acta Anaesthesiologica Scandinavica* 34: 176–182.

5. Cooper J. B., et al. (1984), "An Analysis of Major Errors and Equipment Failures in Anesthesia Management: Considerations for Prevention and Detection," *Anesthesiology* 60: 34–42.

Chapter 3

1. Lundberg, George D., with James Stacey (2000), *Severed Trust* (New York: Basic Books).

2. Roizen, M. F., et al. (2000), in R. D. Miller, ed., *Anesthesia*, 5th ed. (Philadelphia: Churchill Livingstone).

3. Allison, G., and H. R. Bromley (1996), "Unnecessary Preoperative Investigations: Evaluation and Cost Analysis," *American Surgeon* 62: 686–689.

4. Narr, B. J., et al. (1997), "Outcomes of Patients with No Laboratory Assessment Before Anesthesia and a Surgical Procedure," *Mayo Clinic Proceedings* 72: 505–509.

5. Schein, O. D., et al. (2000), *New England Journal of Medicine* 342 (January 20): 168–175.

6. Roizen, M. F., et al. (2000), "Preoperative Evaluation," in R. D. Miller, ed., *Anesthesia*, 5th ed. (Philadelphia: Churchill Livingstone).

7. Starsnic, Mary, et al. (1997), "Efficacy and Financial Benefit of an Anesthesiologist-Directed University Preadmission Evaluation Center," *Journal of Clinical Anesthesia* 9: 299–305.

8. Roizen, et al., "Preoperative Evaluation."

Chapter 4

1. Mendelson, C. L. (1946), "The Aspiration of Stomach Contents Into the Lungs During Obstetric Anesthesia," *American Journal of Obstetrics and Gynecology* 52: 191–205.

2. Cote, C. (1990), "NPO After Midnight for Children—a Reappraisal," *Anesthesiology* 72: 589–591.

3. Warner, M. A., et al. (1999), "Practice Guidelines for Preoperative Fasting and the Use of Pharmacological Agents to Reduce the Risk of Pulmonary Aspiration: Application to Healthy Patients Undergoing Elective Procedures" (a report by the American Society of Anesthesiologists Task Force on Preoperative Fasting) *Anesthesiology* 90: 896–905.

4. Ibid.

Chapter 5

1. McCleane, G., and R. Cooper (1990), "The Nature of Pre-operative Anxiety," *Anesthesia* 45: 153–155.

2. Kain, Z. N., et al. (1997), "Effects of Premedication on Postoperative Behavioral Outcomes in Children," *Anesthesiology* 87: A1032.

3. Ibid.

4. Egbert, L. D., et al. (1963), "The Value of the Preoperative Visit by an Anesthetist," *Journal of the American Medical Association* 185: 553–555.

5. Egbert, L. D., et al. (1964), "Reduction of Postoperative Pain By Encouragement and Instruction of Patients," *New England Journal of Medicine* 270: 825–827.

6. Kain, Z. N., et al. (1999), "Postoperative Behavioral Outcomes in Children: Effects of Sedative Premedication," *Anesthesiology* 90: 758–765.

7. Bowie, Julius (1993), "Parents in the Operating Room," *Anesthesiology* 78: 1192–1193.

8. Kain, Z. N., et al. (1998), "Parental Presence During Induction of Anesthesia Versus Sedative Premedication: Which Is More Effective?" *Anesthesiology* 89: 1147–1156; Kain, Z. N., et al. (2000), "Parental Presence and a Sedative Premedication for Children Undergoing Surgery: A Hierarchical Study," *Anesthesiology* 92: 939–946.

9. Kain, et al. (1998), "Parental Presence During Induction of Anesthesia Versus Sedative Premedication"; Kain, et al. (2000), "Parental Presence and a Sedative Premedication for Children Undergoing Surgery."

Chapter 6

1. Beecher, H. K., and D. P. Todd (1954), "A Study of Deaths Associated with Anesthesia and Surgery," *Annals of Surgery* 14: 2–34; Cohen, M., et al. (1990), "Pediatric Anesthesia Morbidity and Mortality in the Perioperative Period," *Anesthesia and Analgesia* 70: 160–167; Graff, T., et al. (1964), "Baltimore Anesthesia Study Committee: Factors in Pediatric Anesthesia Mortality," *Anesthesia and Analgesia* 43: 407–414; Tiret, L., et al. (1988), "Complications Related to Anaesthesia in Infants and Children: A Prospective Survey of 40,240 Anaesthetics," *British Journal of Anaesthesia* 61: 263–269.

2. Harvey, M. H., et al. (1985), "Inguinal Herniotomy in Children: A Five-Year Survey," *British Journal of Surgery* 72: 485–487; Hotchkiss, W. S. (1960), "Patent Ductus Arteriosus and the Occasional Cardiac Surgeon," *Journal of the American Medical Association* 173: 244–247.

3. Harvey, et al., "Inguinal Herniotomy in Children."

4. Ament, R. (1960), "Classification of Operating Room Mortality: Review of Cases in a Pediatric Medical Center During the 10 Year Period 1949–1958," *Anesthesia and Analgesia* 39: 158–166; Graff, et al., "Baltimore Anesthesia Study Committee."

Chapter 7

1. Merry, A. F., et al. (1992), "First-Time Coronary Artery Bypass Grafting: The Anaesthetist as a Risk Factor," *British Journal of Anesthesia* 68: 6–12; Slogoff, S., and A. S. Keats (1985), "Does Perioperative Myocardial Ischemia Lead to Postoperative Myocardial Infarction?" *Anesthesiology* 62: 107–114.

2. Kennedy, J. W., et al. (1980), Multivariate Discriminant Analysis of the Clinical and Angiographic Predictors of Operative Mortality from the Collaborative Study in Coronary Artery Surgery (CASS)," *Journal of Thoracic and Cardiovascular Surgery* 80: 876–887; Luft, H. S., et al. (1979), "Should

Operations Be Regionalized? The Empirical Relationship Between Surgical Volume and Mortality," *New England Journal of Medicine* 301: 1364–1369; Luft, H. S. (1980), "The Relation Between Surgical Volume and Mortality: An Exploration of Causal Factors and Alternative Models," *Medical Care* 18: 940–959.

Chapter 8

1. Saklad, M. (1941), "Grading of Patients for Surgical Procedures," *Anesthesiology* 2: 281–284.
2. Cohen, M. M., and P. G. Duncan (1988), "Physical Status Score and Trends in Complications," *Journal of Clinical Epidemiology* 41: 83–90; Pederson, T., et al. (1990), "A Prospective Study of Mortality Associated with Anaesthesia and Surgery: Risk Indicators of Mortality in Hospital," *Acta Anaesthesiologica Scandinavica* 34: 176–182; Tiret, L., and F. Hatton (1986), "Complications Associated with Anaesthesia—A Prospective Survey in France," *Canadian Anaesthetists' Society Journal* 33: 336–344; Vacanti, C. J., et al. (1970), "A Statistical Analysis of the Relationship of Physical Status to Postoperative Mortality in 68,388 Cases," *Anesthesia and Analgesia* 49: 564–566.

Chapter 9

1. Denborough, M. A., and R. R. Lovell (1960), "Anesthetic Deaths in a Family," *Lancet* 2: 45.
2. Gravenstein, N., and R. R. Kirby, eds. (1996), *Complications in Anesthesiology: Malignant Hyperthermia*, 2nd ed. (Philadelphia: Lippincott-Raven), pp. 141–162.

Chapter 10

1. Brody, G. L., and R. B. Sweet (1963), "Halothane As a Possible Cause of Massive Hepatic Necrosis," *Anesthesiology* 24: 29–37; Bunker, J. P., and C. M. Blumenfeld (1963), "Liver Necrosis After Halothane Anesthesia," *New England Journal of Medicine* 268: 531–534; Lindenbaum, J., and E. Leifer

(1963), "Hepatic Necrosis Associated with Halothane Anesthesia," *New England Journal of Medicine* 268: 525.

2. Bunker, J. P., et al. (1966), "Summary of the National Halothane Study: Possible Association Between Halothane Anesthesia and Post-Operative Hepatic Necrosis," *Journal of the American Medical Association* 197: 121–134.

3. Ibid.

4. Ibid.

Chapter 11

1. Green, R. A. (1986), "A Matter of Vigilance," *Anaesthesia* 40: 129–130.

2. American Society of Anesthesiologists (1999), "ASA Standards for Basic Anesthetic Monitoring," in *ASA Directory of Members* (Park Ridge, IL: ASA), pp. 462–463.

3. Cooper, J. B., et al. (1984), "An Analysis of Major Errors and Equipment Failures in Anesthesia Management: Considerations for Prevention and Detection," *Anesthesiology* 60: 34–42; Cooper, J. B., et al. (1982), "Critical Incidents Associated with Intraoperative Exchanges of Anesthesia Personnel," *Anesthesiology* 56: 456–461; Cooper, J. B., et al. (1978), "Preventable Anesthesia Mishaps: A Study of Human Factors," *Anesthesiology* 49: 399–406; Gaba, D. M., et al. (1987), "Anesthetic Mishaps: Breaking the Chain of Accident Evolution," *Anesthesiology* 66: 670–676; Kumar, V., et al. (1988), "An Analysis of Critical Incidents in a Teaching Department for Quality Assurance: A Survey of Mishaps During Anaesthesia," *Anaesthesia* 43: 879–883.

4. Allnutt, M. F. (1987), "Human Factors in Accidents," *British Journal of Anaesthesia* 59: 856–864; Gaba D. M. (1989), "Human Error in Anesthetic Mishaps," *International Anesthesiology Clinics* 17: 137–147; Gaba, et al., "Anesthetic Mishaps: Breaking the Chain."

5. Cooper, J. B. (1988), "Do Short Breaks Increase or Decrease Anesthetic Risk?" *Journal of Clinical Anesthesia* 1: 228–231; Cooper, et al. (1984), "An Analysis of Major Errors and Equipment Failures."

6. Dawson, D., and K. Reid (1997), "Fatigue, Alcohol, and Performance Impairment," *Nature* 388: 235.

Chapter 12

1. Fenster, Julie M. (2001), *Ether Day* (New York: HarperCollins).

2. Cooper, J. B., et al. (1984), "An Analysis of Major Errors and Equipment Failures in Anesthesia Management: Considerations for Prevention and Detection," *Anesthesiology* 60: 34–42.

3. Cooper, J. B., et al. (1978), "Preventable Anesthesia Mishaps: A Study of Human Factors," *Anesthesiology* 49: 399–406.

Chapter 14

1. American Society of Anesthesiologists (1999), "ASA Standards for Basic Anesthetic Monitoring," in *ASA Directory of Members* (Park Ridge, IL: ASA), pp. 462–463.

2. Ibid.

3. Caplan, R. A., et al. (1990), "Adverse Respiratory Events in Anesthesia: A Closed Claims Analysis," *Anesthesiology* 72: 828–833; Tinker, J. H., et al. (1989), "Role of Monitoring Devices in Prevention of Anesthetic Mishaps: A Closed Claim Analysis," *Anesthesiology* 71: 541–546; Eichhorn, J. H. (1989), "Prevention of Intraoperative Anesthesia Accidents and Related Severe Injury Through Safety Monitoring," *Anesthesiology* 70: 572–577.

Chapter 15

1. Griffith, H. R., and G. E. Johnson (1942), "The Use of Curare in General Anesthesia," *Anesthesiology* 3: 418–420.

Chapter 16

1. McCleane, G. J., and R. Cooper (1990), "The Nature of Pre-operative Anxiety," *Anaesthesia* 45: 153–155.

2. Liu, W.H.D., et al. (1991), "Incidence of Awareness with Recall During General Anesthesia," *Anaesthesia* 46: 435–437.

3. Lyons, G., and R. MacDonald (1991), "Awareness During Caesarean Section," *Anaesthesia* 46: 62–64.

4. Phillips, A. A., et al. (1993), "Recall of Intraoperative Events After

General Anaesthesia and Cardiopulmonary Bypass," *Canadian Journal of Anaesthesia* 40: 922–926.

5. Bogetz, M. S., and J. A. Katz (1984), "Recall of Surgery for Major Trauma," *Anesthesiology* 61: 6–9.

6. Crawford, J. S. (1971), "Awareness During Operative Obstetrics Under General Anesthesia," *British Journal of Anaesthesia* 43: 179–182; Domino, K. B., et al. (1999), "Awareness During Anesthesia: A Closed Claims Analysis," *Anesthesiology* 90: 1053–1061; Schwender, D., et al. (1998), "Conscious Awareness During General Anesthesia: Patient's Perceptions, Emotions, Cognition and Reactions," *British Journal of Anaesthesia* 80: 133–139.

7. Blacher, R. S. (1975), "On Awakening Paralyzed During Surgery: A Syndrome of Traumatic Neurosis," *Journal of the American Medical Association* 234: 67–68; Schwender, et al., "Conscious Awareness During General Anesthesia."

8. Blacher, "On Awakening Paralyzed During Surgery."

9. Aitkenhead, A. R. (1990), "Awareness During Anaesthesia: What Should the Patient Be Told?" *Anaesthesia* 45: 351–352.

10. Domino, et al., "Awareness During Anesthesia."

11. Ibid.

12. Bogetz and Katz, "Recall of Surgery."

13. Phillips, et al., "Recall of Intraoperative Events."

14. Crawford, "Awareness During Operative Obstetrics"; Lyons and MacDonald, "Awareness During Caesarean Section."

15. Aitkenhead, "Awareness During Anaesthesia."

16. Ibid.

17. Lyons and MacDonald, "Awareness During Caesarean Section."

18. Sebel, P. S. (2001), "Can We Monitor Depth of Anesthesia?" 2001 International Anesthesia Research Society Review Course Lectures.

Chapter 17

1. Domino, K. B., et al. (1999), "Awareness During Anesthesia: A Closed Claims Analysis," *Anesthesiology* 90: 1053–1061.

2. Johansen, J. W., and P. S. Sebel (2000), "Development and Clinical Application of Electroencephalographic Bispectrum Monitoring,"

Anesthesiology 93: 1336–1344; Sebel, P. S. (2001), "Can We Monitor Depth of Anesthesia?" 2001 International Anesthesia Research Society Review Course Lectures.

3. Glass, P. S., et al. (1997), "Bispectral Analysis Measures Sedation and Memory Effects of Propofol, Midazolam, Isoflurane, and Alfentanil in Healthy Volunteers," *Anesthesiology* 86: 836–847.

4. Ibid.; Sebel, "Can We Monitor Depth of Anesthesia?"

5. Sebel, "Can We Monitor Depth of Anesthesia?"

Chapter 18

1. Bedford, P. D. (1955), "Adverse Cerebral Effects of Anaesthesia on Old People," *Lancet* 2: 257–263.

2. Knill, R. L., et al. (1991), "Idiopathic Postoperative Delirium Is Associated with Long-Term Cognitive Impairment," *Canadian Journal of Anesthesia* 38: A54; Moller, J. T., et al. (1998), "Long-Term Postoperative Cognitive Dysfunction in the Elderly: ISPOCD1 Study," *Lancet* 351: 857–861.

3. Knill, et al., "Idiopathic Postoperative Delirium."

4. Moller, et al., "Long-Term Postoperative Cognitive Dysfunction."

5. Francis, J., et al. (1990), "A Prospective Study of Delirium in Hospitalized Elderly," *Journal of the American Medical Association* 263: 1097–1101; Rockwood, K. (1989), "Acute Confusion in Elderly Medical Patients," *Journal of the American Geriatric Society* 37: 150–154.

6. Williams-Russo, P., et al. (1995), "Cognitive Effects After Epidural Versus General Anesthesia in Older Adults," *Journal of the American Medical Association* 274: 44–50.

7. Parikh, S. S., and F. Chung (1995), "Postoperative Delerium in the Elderly," *Anesthesia and Analgesia* 80: 1223–1232.

8. Gustafson, Y., et al. (1991), "A Geriatric Anesthesiologic Program to Reduce Acute Confusional States in Elderly Patients Treated for Femoral Neck Fractures," *Journal of American Geriatric Society* 39: 655–662.

9. Ibid.

Chapter 19

1. Derrington, M. C., and G. Smith (1987), "A Review of Studies of Anaesthetic Risk, Morbidity, and Mortality," *British Journal of Anaesthesia* 59: 815–833.

2. Beecher, H. K., and D. P. Todd (1954), "A Study of Deaths Associated with Anesthesia and Surgery," *Annals of Surgery* 14: 2–34.

3. Buck, N., et al. (1987), *The Report of a Confidential Enquiry Into Perioperative Deaths (CEPOD)* (London: Nuffield Provincial Hospitals Trust).

4. Warden, J. C., and B. F. Horan (1996), "Deaths Attributed to Anaesthesia in New South Wales, 1984–1990," *Anaesthesia and Intensive Care* 24: 66–73.

5. Eichhorn, J. H. (1989), "Prevention of Intraoperative Anesthesia Accidents and Related Severe Injury Through Safety Monitoring," *Anesthesiology* 70: 572–577.

6. Ibid.

7. Ibid.

8. Kennedy, J. W., et al. (1980), "Multivariate Discriminant Analysis of the Clinical and Angiographic Predictors of Operative Mortality from the Collaborative Study in Coronary Artery Surgery (CASS)," *Journal of Thoracic and Cardiovascular Surgery* 80: 876–887; Luft, H. S., et al. (1979), "Should Operations Be Regionalized? The Empirical Relationship Between Surgical Volume and Mortality," *New England Journal of Medicine* 301: 1364–1369.

9. Kennedy, et al. "Multivariate Discriminant Analysis"; Luft, H. S., et al. (1980), "The Empirical Relation Between Surgical Volume and Mortality: An Exploration of Causal Factors and Alternative Models," *Medical Care* 18: 940–959.

10. Harvey, M. H., et al. (1985), "Inguinal Herniotomy in Children: A Five-Year Survey," *British Journal of Surgery* 72:485–487.

11. Hotchkiss, W. S. (1960), "Patent Ductus Arteriosus and the Occasional Cardiac Surgeon," *Journal of the American Medical Association* 173: 244–247.

12. Bechtoldt, A. A. Jr. (1981), "Committee on Anesthesia Study: Anesthetic-Related Deaths, 1969–1976," *North Carolina Medical Journal* 42: 253–259; Forrest, W.H. (1980), "Outcome: The Effect of the Provider," in R. A. Hirsh, et al., eds., *Health Care Delivery in Anesthesia* (Philadelphia: George F.

Stickley), pp. 137–142; Holland, R. (1987), "Anaesthetic Mortality in New South Wales," *British Journal of Anaesthesia* 59: 834–841.

Chapter 20

1. Pederson T., and S. H. Johansen (1989), "Serious Morbidity Attributable to Anaesthesia: Considerations for Prevention," *Anaesthesia* 44: 504–508.

2. Tiret, L., and F. Hatton (1986), "Complications Associated with Anaesthesia-A Prospective Survey in France," *Canadian Anaesthetists' Society Joutnal* 33: 336–344.

3. Kroll, D., et al. (1990), "Nerve Injury Associated with Anesthesia," *Anesthesiology* 73: 202–207.

Chapter 21

1. Duncan, P. G., and M. M. Cohen (1987), "Postoperative Complications: Factors of Significance to Anaesthesia Practice," *Canadian Journal of Anaesthesia* 34: 2–8; Hines, R., et al. (1992), "Complications Occurring in the Postanesthesia Care Unit: A Survey," *Anesthesia and Analgesia* 74: 503–509; Tiret, L., and F. Hatton (1986), "Complications Associated with Anaesthesia-A Prospective Survey in France," *Canadian Anaesthetists' Society Journal* 33: 336–344; Tiret L., et al. (1988), "Complications Related to Anaesthesia in Infants and Children: A Prospective Survey of 40,240 Anaesthetics," *British Journal of Anaesthesia* 61: 263–269.

2. Tiret and Hatton, "Complications Associated with Anaesthesia."

3. Warden, J. C., and B. F. Horan (1996), "Deaths Attributed to Anaesthesia in New South Wales, 1984–1990," *Anaesthesia and Intensive Care* 24: 66–73.

4. Duncan and Cohen, "Postoperative Complications."

5. Tiret and Hatton, "Complications Associated with Anaesthesia."

6. American Society of Anesthesiologists (1996), "Standards for Postanesthesia Care," in *Directory of Members* (Park Ridge, IL: ASA), p. 395.

Chapter 22

1. McCleane, G. J., and R. Cooper (1990), "The Nature of Preoperative Anxiety," *Anaesthesia* 45: 153–155.

2. Fujii, Y., et al. (1995), "Granesitron-Dexamethasone Combination Reduces Postoperative Nausea and Vomiting," *Canadian Journal of Anaesthesia* 42: 387.

Chapter 23

1. Hill, C. S. Jr. (1991), *New Strategies in Pain Management* (newsletter), Report on a Symposium, *Eighth International Congress on Care of the Terminally Ill* (Whippany, NJ: Knoll Pharmaceuticals); McGrath, P. J., and G. Frager (1996), "Psychological Barriers to Optimal Pain Management in Infants and Children," *Clinical Journal of Pain* 12: 135–141; Porter, J., and H. Hick (1980), "Addiction Rare in Patients Treated with Narcotics," *New England Journal of Medicine* 302: 123.

2. Hill, *New Strategies in Pain Management.*

3. Ibid.; McGrath and Frager, "Psychological Barriers to Optimal Pain Management"; Porter and Hick, "Addiction Rare in Patients Treated with Narcotics."

Chapter 24

1. Egbert, L. D., et al. (1964), "Reduction of Postoperative Pain By Encouragement and Instruction of Patients," *New England Journal of Medicine* 270: 825–827.

2. Ferrante, F. M., et al. (1990), *Patient Controlled Analgesia* (Boston: Blackwell Scientific).

3. Cousins, M. J., and L. E. Mather (1984), "Intrathecal and Epidural Administration of Opioids," *Anesthesiology* 61: 276–310; Ferrante, F. M. (1998), "Acute Postoperative Pain Management," in D. E. Longnecker, et al., eds., *Principles and Practice of Anesthesiology*, 2nd ed. (St. Louis: Mosby); Ready, L.B. (2000), "Acute Perioperative Pain," in R. D. Miller, ed., *Anesthesia*, 5th ed. (Philadelphia: Churchill Livingstone).

4. Cousins and Mather, "Intrathecal and Epidural Administration of Opioids."

5. Kehlet, H., and J. B. Dahl (1993), "The Value of 'Multimodal' or 'Balanced Analgesia' in Postoperative Pain Treatment," *Anesthesia and Analgesia* 77: 1048–1056.

Chapter 25

1. Cote, C. J., et al. (2000), "Adverse Sedation Events in Pediatrics: A Critical Incident Analysis of Contributory Factors," *Pediatrics* 105: 805–814; Cote, C. J., et al. (2000), "Adverse Sedation Events in Pediatrics: Analysis of Medications Used for Sedation," *Pediatrics* 106: 633–644.

2. Courtiss, E. H., et al. (1994), "Anesthetic Practices in Ambulatory Aesthetic Surgery," *Plastic and Reconstructive Surgery* 93: 792–801.

3. Malviya S., et al. (1997), "Adverse Events and Risk Factors Associated with the Sedation of Children By Non-Anesthesiologists," *Anesthesia and Analgesia* 85: 1207–1213.

4. Keeter, S., et al. (1990), "Sedation in Pediatric CT: National Survey of Current Practice," *Radiology* 175: 745–752; Morton, N. S., and G. J. Oomen (1998), "Development of a Selection and Monitoring Protocol for Safe Sedation of Children," *Paediatric Anaesthesia* 8: 65–68.

5. Cote, C. J., et al., "Adverse Sedation Events in Pediatrics: A Critical Incident Analysis"; Cote, C. J., et al. (2000), "Adverse Sedation Events in Pediatrics: Analysis of Medications."

6. Cote, C. J., et al., "Adverse Sedation Events in Pediatrics: A Critical Incident Analysis"; Cote, C. J., et al., "Adverse Sedation Events in Pediatrics: Analysis of Medications."

7. Cote, C. J., et al., "Adverse Sedation Events in Pediatrics: A Critical Incident Analysis"; Cote, C. J., et al., "Adverse Sedation Events in Pediatrics: Analysis of Medications."

8. Cote, C. J., et al., "Adverse Sedation Events in Pediatrics: A Critical Incident Analysis"; Cote, et al., "Adverse Sedation Events in Pediatrics: Analysis of Medications."

9. Cote, C. J., et al., "Adverse Sedation Events in Pediatrics: A Critical Incident Analysis"; Cote, C. J., et al., "Adverse Sedation Events in Pediatrics: Analysis of Medications."

10. Cote, C. J., et al., "Adverse Sedation Events in Pediatrics: A Critical Incident Analysis"; Cote, C. J., et al., "Adverse Sedation Events in Pediatrics: Analysis of Medications."

11. American Academy of Pediatrics, Committee on Drugs (1992), "Guidelines for Monitoring and Management of Pediatric Patients During and After Sedation for Diagnostic and Therapeutic Procedures," *Pediatrics* 89: 1110–1115.

Chapter 26

1. Hutter, C. D. (1990), "The Wooley and Roe Case," *Anaesthesia* 45: 859–864; Kennedy, F., et al. (1950), "The Grave Spinal Cord Paralyses Caused By Spinal Anesthesia," *Surgery, Gynecology, and Obstetrics* 91: 385–398.

2. Ibid.

3. Marinacci, A. A. (1960), "Neurological Aspects of Complications of Spinal Anesthesia," *Los Angeles Neurological Society Bulletin* 25: 170.

4. Vandam, L. D., and R. D. Dripps (1955), "A Long-Term Follow-Up of Patients Who Received 10,098 Spinal Anesthetics, II: Incidence and Analysis of Minor Sensory Neurological Defects," *Surgery* 38: 463–469.

5. Moore, D. C., and L. D. Bridenbaugh (1966), "Spinal (Subarachnoid) Block: A Review of 11,574 Cases," *Journal of the American Medical Association* 195: 907–912.

6. Kane, R. E. (1981), "Neurological Deficits Following Epidural or Spinal Anesthesia," *Anesthesia and Analgesia* 60: 150–161.

7. Caplan, R. A., et al. (1988), "Unexpected Cardiac Arrest During Spinal Anesthesia: A Closed Claim Analysis of Predisposing Factors," *Anesthesiology* 68: 5–11.

Chapter 27

1. Kehlet, H., and J. B. Dahl (1993), "The Value of 'Multimodal' or 'Balanced Analgesia' in Postoperative Pain Treatment," *Anesthesia and Analgesia* 77: 1048–1056; Liu, S., et al. (1995), "Epidural Anesthesia and Analgesia: Their Role in Postoperative Outcome," *Anesthesiology* 82: 1474–1506.

2. Kehlet, H. (1998), "General Versus Regional Anesthesia," in D. E. Longnecker, et al., eds., *Principles and Practice of Anesthesiology*, 2nd ed. (St. Louis: Mosby); Liu, et al., "Epidural Anesthesia and Analgesia."

3. Ibid.; Riis, J., et al. (1983), "Immediate and Long-Term Mental Recovery from General Versus Epidural Anesthesia in Elderly Patients," *Acta Anaesthesiologica Scandinavica* 27: 44–49; Williams-Russo, P., et al. (1995), "Cognitive Effects After Epidural Versus General Anesthesia in Older Adults," *Journal of the American Medical Association* 274: 44–50.

4. Bode, R. H., et al. (1996), "Cardiac Outcome After Peripheral Vascular Surgery: Comparison of General and Regional Anesthesia," *Anesthesiology* 84: 3–13; Christopherson, R., et al. (1993), "Perioperative Morbidity in Patients Randomized to Epidural or General Anesthesia for Lower Extremity Vascular Surgery," *Anesthesiology* 79: 422–434; Liu, et al., "Epidural Anesthesia and Analgesia"; Williams-Russo, et al., "Cognitive Effects."

Chapter 28

1. Koch M. E. (1999), "Considerations in Office-Based Anesthesia," American Society of Anesthesiologists Refresher Course Lecture 216 (Park Ridge, IL: ASA).

2. Morrell, R. C. (2000), "OBA Questions, Problems Just Now Recognized," *Anesthesia Patient Safety Foundation Newsletter* 15: 1–3.

3. Courtiss, E. H., et al. (1994), "Anesthetic Practices in Ambulatory Aesthetic Surgery," *Plastic and Reconstructive Surgery* 93: 792–801.

4. Cote, C. J., et al. (2000), "Adverse Sedation Events in Pediatrics: A Critical Incident Analysis of Contributory Factors," *Pediatrics* 105: 805–814.

5. Courtiss, et al., "Anesthetic Practices."

6. Morrell, "OBA Questions."

7. Stoelting, R. K. (2000), "Anesthesia Patient Safety Foundation Provides Guidance to Public, Patients: Questions to Ask Before Accepting Office-Based Anesthesia," *Anesthesia Patient Safety Foundation Newsletter*.

8. Ibid.

INDEX